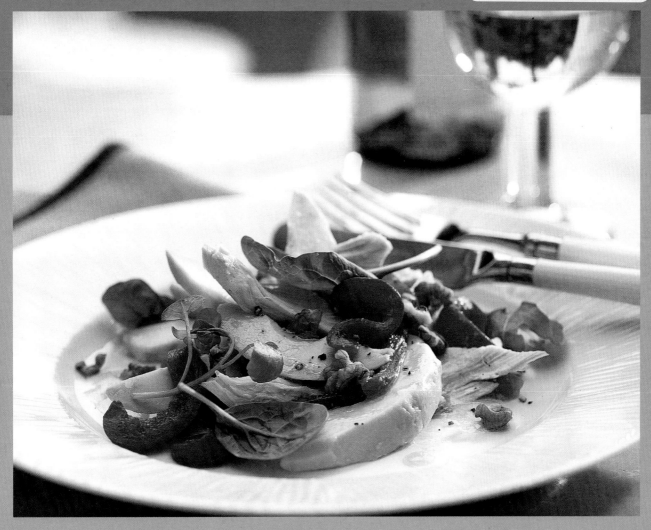

GREAT **HEALTHY** FOOD

DIABETES

AZMINA GOVINDJI

FIREFLY BOOKS

A FIREFLY BOOK

Published by Firefly Books Ltd., 2003

National Library of Canada Cataloguing in Publication
Govindji, Azmina
   Great healthy food for diabetes / Azmina Govindji.
Includes index.
ISBN 1-55297-651-3
1. Diabetes—Diet therapy—Recipes. 2. Diabetes—Diet therapy. I. Title.
RC662.G69 2003   641.5'6314   C2002-902730-6

Publisher Cataloging-in-Publication Data
(Library of Congress Standards)
Giovindji, Azmina.
   Great Healthy Food for Diabetes / Azmina Giovindji. – 1st ed.
[128] p. : col. ill. : photos. ;   cm.
Includes index.
ISBN 1-55297-651-3
1. Diabetes – Diet therapy – Recipes. 2. Diabetes – Nutritional aspects. 3. Diabetic Diet. I. Title.   616.4/ 620654   21 RC662.G56 2003

Published in the United States in 2003 by Firefly Books (U.S.) Inc.
P.O. Box 1338, Ellicott Station
Buffalo, New York 14205

First published in Canada in 2003 by Firefly Books Ltd.
3680 Victoria Park Avenue
Toronto, Ontario M2H 3K1

Reproduced by Colourscan, Singapore
Printed and bound in Great Britain by The Bath Press

Not all the recipes in this cookbook are necessarily appropriate for all people with diabetes. Health care providers and dietitians can help design specific meal plans.

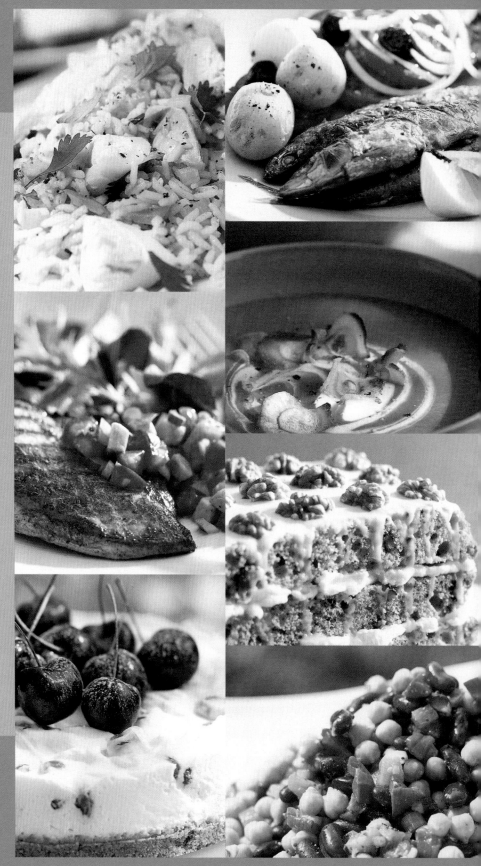

Contents

Introduction

Eating is one of the great pleasures of life, and there's no reason to miss out if you have diabetes. You can still enjoy an array of appetizing and mouth-watering flavors and aromas, while making healthy choices for you and your family. This book will show you what you *can* eat, not give you a list of those foods you should avoid. The recipes are delicious and varied—you'll come across delights such as Monkfish Kabobs with Lemon and Thyme, and Turkey with Red Onion and Watercress Salad, along with traditional favorites like Stuffed Peppers. You also can treat yourself with the Chocolate and Almond Custard Tart or the Banana Ice Cream with Chocolate and Hazelnut Topping.

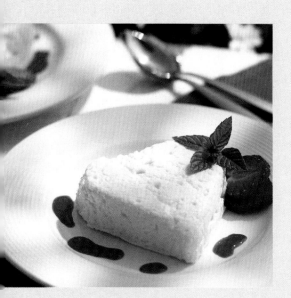

WHAT THIS BOOK OFFERS

Each recipe featured in the book has been carefully tested using the latest guidelines for a diabetes meal plan—all of the meals and snacks combine a range of appropriate ingredients that help you to maintain steady glucose levels. Healthy eating, particularly for people with diabetes, is all about balance. It's also about being able to choose a variety of foods you enjoy and making them part of a healthy lifestyle that fits in with your current food preferences and eating habits—you don't need to completely change your diet.

Many of the recipes are based on the tempting tastes of the Mediterranean. Foods such as fatty fish, garlic, olive oil, fruit and vegetables all play a part in the healthy Mediterranean diet, which research studies have found to have significant health benefits for people with diabetes. The recipes in this book have been specifically created so that you get the best out of these ingredients.

Some of the dishes featured in this book may, at first, appear to be absolute foods to avoid for people with diabetes. But let's dispel the myth that people with diabetes need a special diet. All foods can be incorporated into a healthy way of eating—it's getting the combinations right that's important. Rich chocolate desserts and main meals cooked in butter may sound totally out of the question, but remember that the recipes in this book have been created in line with healthy eating principles and generally use low-fat, low-calorie ingredients, such as reduced-fat spreads, low-fat yogurt, and so on.

Each chapter in this book contains recipes for meals that will be enjoyed by family and friends, whether or not they have diabetes. You'll also notice some magnificent ideas for entertaining, so you can be sure that you're looking after your diet even when you're having fun with friends. Throughout, I've given recipe variations so you can enjoy different, yet equally delicious, creations as you desire.

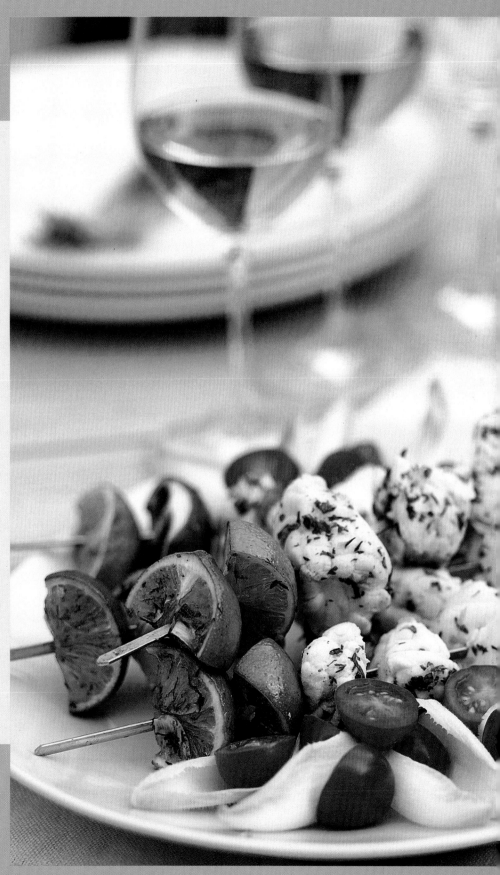

WHAT IS DIABETES?

When you have diabetes, the amount of glucose in your blood is too high. Insulin, the hormone that helps glucose enter the cells where it is used as fuel by the body, is not produced in sufficient quantities by a person with diabetes. If there is not enough insulin, or if the insulin you have is not working well, then glucose can build up in your blood. This causes the symptoms of diabetes, which are excessive thirst, a dry mouth, passing large amounts of urine, loss of weight, tiredness, itchy skin and blurred vision.

There are two kinds of diabetes: **Non-insulin-dependent diabetes** is the most common type. The body can still make some insulin, but not enough for its needs. Non-insulin-dependent diabetes can usually be treated by a healthy diet alone plus physical activity; or by a combination of diet, activity and tablets; or by diet, activity and insulin injections. **Insulin-dependent diabetes** occurs when the body is unable to produce its own insulin. It is treated with insulin injections, combined with a healthy diet and regular activity.

One main goal of management is to avoid highs and lows in the body's blood glucose level. Together with a healthy lifestyle, this will help to improve your well-being and protect against long-term damage to your eyes, kidneys, nerves and heart. There is no cure for diabetes, but with the proper management, you can enjoy a full, healthy and active life.

NUTRITIONAL GUIDELINES

Eat regular meals – this will help your blood glucose remain steady throughout the day.

Try to get to a healthy weight and stay there—being overweight can put a strain on your body organs, especially the heart.

Select foods with a low glycemic index—the latest research highlights the theory of Glycemic Index (GI), which ranks foods according to how they affect blood glucose levels. The faster a food is broken down during digestion, the quicker blood glucose levels will rise. Foods that cause a rapid rise in blood glucose will have a high GI, so choose more foods with low GIs regularly. Foods that are high in soluble fiber, such as whole-grain, pumpernickel and rye bread, peas, corn, beans, lentils, citrus fruits and oats, have a low GI.

Make starchy foods (such as bread, potatoes, pasta, cereals and rice) the main part of your meal—starchy carbohydrates will help to fill you up, and tend to be lower in calories than processed foods containing more fat.

Cut down on fried and higher-fat foods, such as butter, regular cheese, fatty meats, donuts and pastries—fats are an essential component of the diet, but too many saturated fats, found in meat and dairy products, can lead to a build-up of fat in the arteries, which can reduce blood flow to the heart.

Eat five portions of fruit and vegetables a day—fruit and vegetables contain vital antioxidant vitamins (A, C and E). Antioxidants protect against free radicals, which, though formed naturally by the body, can cause damage and increase your risks of cardiovascular disease.

Swap high-sugar foods (e.g. canned fruit in syrup) for low-sugar foods (e.g. canned fruit in natural juice)—high-sugar foods cause glucose levels to rise quickly, so it is important to keep an eye on your sugar intake. It is, however, a misconception that people with diabetes should avoid sugar altogether. High-sugar foods and drinks, consumed alone, can rapidly increase blood glucose. However, if sugar is eaten with other foods, especially at the end of a high-fiber meal, the blood glucose rises more slowly, as this increases the time it takes for the sugar to enter the bloodstream.

Eat more fish and have fatty fish once a week—scientific studies suggest that fatty fish may be protective against heart problems. Omega-3 oils, found in fatty fish, have been shown to lower blood fats like cholesterol.

Choose foods that are low in salt—eating too much salt has been associated with high blood pressure and stroke. Most of the salt you eat comes from processed foods, such as bacon, canned foods and salted snack foods. Choose home-prepared foods where you have control over the amount of salt added.

THE IMPORTANCE OF DIET

What you eat is the most important part of any treatment for diabetes. Whether you need to take medication or not, the foods you choose and how often you eat have a significant effect on your blood glucose levels—watching your meal plan allows you to control the level of glucose in your blood. A low saturated fat diet is particularly beneficial for people with diabetes, who have an increased risk of developing heart disease. Remember that insulin or tablets are not a substitute for a healthy diet.

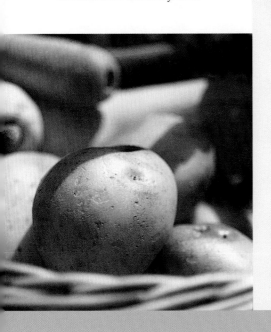

Chapter 1 helps you start the day with inspiring choices for breakfast, featuring recipes containing high-fiber ingredients such as oats and fruit, as well as egg dishes. Breakfast is a very important meal for people with diabetes to help control blood glucose levels.

In Chapter 2, you'll find a collection of light meals and snacks, including sandwiches, salads, stuffed potatoes and pizza. It is often recommended that people with diabetes spread their carbohydrates out over the day, so these recipes are ideal choices for food that can be eaten throughout the day. This chapter also introduces you to different breads, for example ciabatta and pita, as well as giving away tricks of the trade, such as a lower-fat way of making popcorn.

Chapter 3 paves the way for the main meals to follow, featuring a varied selection of appetizers and soups, perfect for entertaining. These recipes have been created to release glucose into the bloodstream gradually, and to help avoid blood glucose levels from rising too high after meals.

You can afford to be adventurous with the meat, fish, poultry and vegetarian main courses in Chapter 4, as you'll be given step-by-step instructions in all the recipes, which include risottos, stir-fries and even home-made wraps. Cooking methods such as baking, pan-frying, grilling and boiling all go a long way to ensure that you keep the fat low, while preserving all the natural flavors and goodness of the carefully selected ingredients. This chapter also contains useful tips on starchy foods, such as polenta and couscous, allowing you to increase your repertoire for filling and tasty meals.

Chapter 5 presents you with ideas for many colorful vegetable dishes, along with many other accompaniments, which include beans, legumes and traditional Mediterranean favorites. Vegetables are a crucial part of a healthy meal plan, as they provide essential vitamins and minerals and are high in

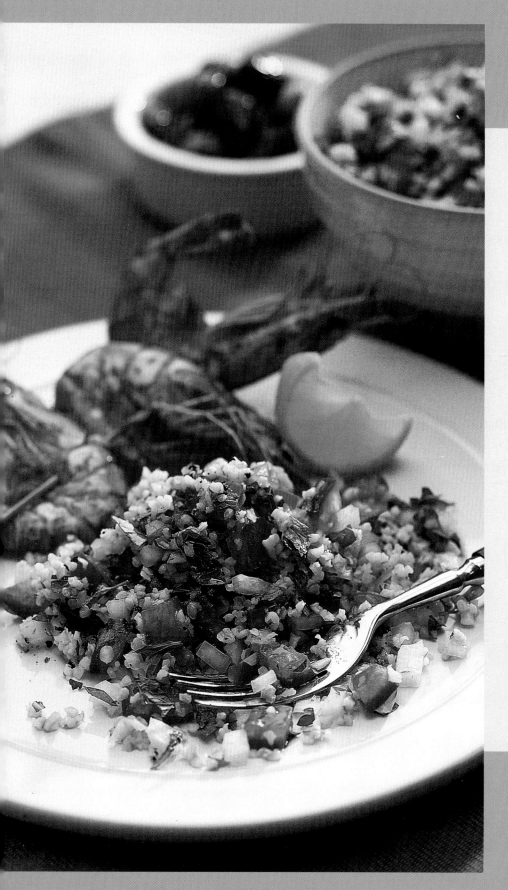

fiber, which fills you up, helping to prevent weight gain—this is an important consideration for many people with diabetes.

Chapter 6 demonstrates that people with diabetes can enjoy a wide variety of delicious desserts, while maintaining a healthy diet. The hot, cold and iced desserts are oozing with ingredients like fresh raspberries, almonds, chocolate, lime, cinnamon, ginger and much more.

The cakes and breads in Chapter 7 will inspire you with quick and easy ways to conjure up your own treats for a special occasion or snack. This chapter includes recipes for whole-grain bread, fruit scones and flapjacks, as well as a range of cakes and crunchy treats.

The recipes in this book demonstrate that a diabetes meal plan need not be limited. Food for diabetes is all about the enjoyment of delicious ingredients and an appreciation of healthy eating. With quality

Mediterranean ingredients combined in inventive, creative recipes that use healthy cooking methods, this book is your chance to have your cake and eat it, whether you have diabetes or not!

Notes to the Cook

Most of the ingredients in this book will be available from your local supermarket or grocery store. To help you watch your fat intake, I've suggested using ingredients such as cooking spray, low-fat sour cream or reduced-fat margarines. Regular margarines are used in some recipes as reduced-fat margarines contain too much water to produce quality results. It is therefore important to note which type of fat is listed in the ingredients. Where a recipe calls for salt, use the minimum possible and for pepper, choose freshly ground black pepper.

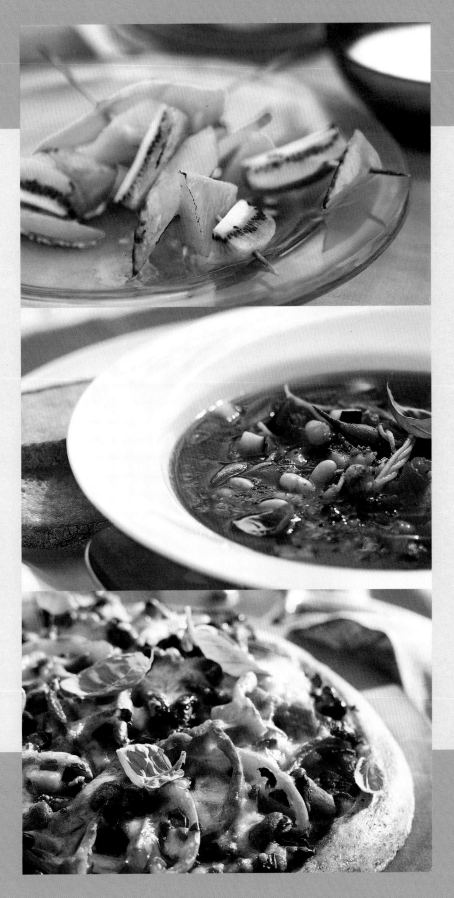

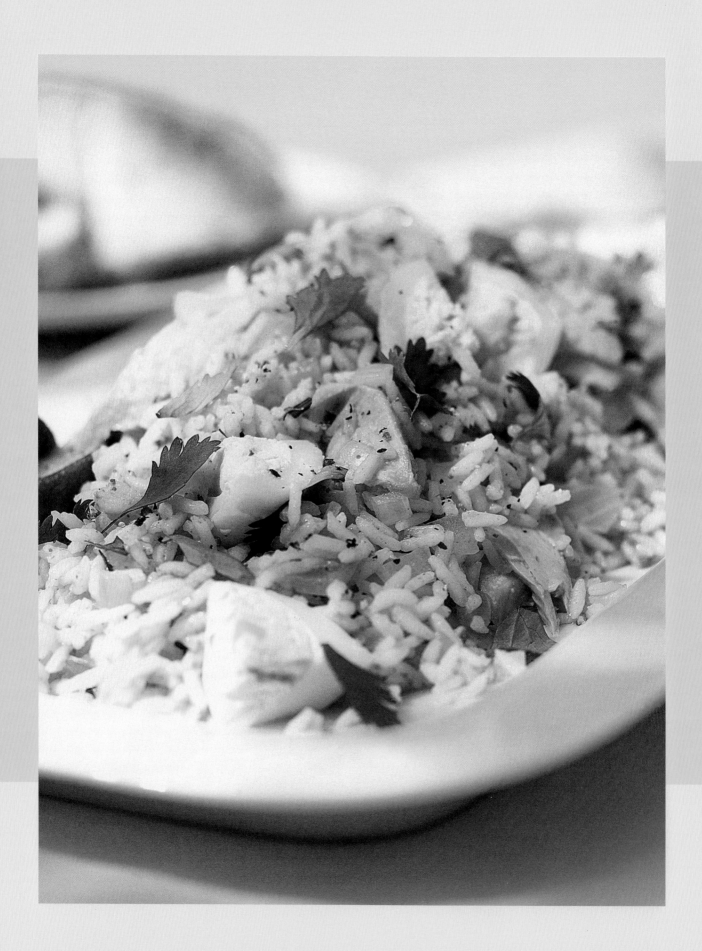

Breakfasts

1

GRAINS & CEREALS

FRUIT

EGGS, FISH & CHEESE

VEGETABLES

OATMEAL COOKIES WITH RAISINS & SOUR CHERRIES

Instead of buying expensive granola bars, try these moist, fruity cookies, which can be warmed up in the oven or microwave. There is unlikely to be a healthier way to start your day.

½ cup (125 ml) butter

¾ cup (175 ml) light brown sugar

1 cup (250 ml) self-rising flour

Pinch of salt

1½ cups (375 ml) rolled or quick-cooking oats

1 large egg, beaten

⅔ cup (150 ml) skim milk

1 cup (250 ml) dried sour cherries

1 cup (250 ml) raisins

Makes 25–30 cookies

1 Preheat the oven to 350°F (180°C). In a large mixing bowl, cream the butter and sugar together, then mix in the flour, salt and oats.

2 Add the beaten egg and most of the milk until the mixture is stiff—you may not need to add all the milk. Mix thoroughly, and fold in the dried fruit. Give it a final mix.

3 Using a teaspoon, place walnut-size pieces of dough onto a non-stick baking sheet (the mixture spreads only slightly, so they do not need to be too far apart).

4 Bake in the oven for about 20 minutes or until golden brown.

HOMEMADE CRUNCHY MUESLI

This luxury muesli is a satisfying mix of sweet, golden apricots, sunflower seeds and crunchy chopped pecans in an oat base. Serve with low fat milk, berries, slices of fresh fruit and a swirl of low-fat yogurt.

4 cups (1 liter) quick oats

½ cup (125 ml) toasted sunflower seeds

1⅓ cup (325 ml) seedless raisins

½ cup (125 ml) chopped pecans

⅓ cup (75 ml) dried apricots, chopped

Makes 14 servings

1 Mix all the ingredients together thoroughly, and transfer the muesli to an airtight container to store.

2 To serve, spoon into a serving bowl, pour over some 2% milk and add slices of your favorite fresh fruit and a creamy topping such as low-fat yogurt or sour cream.

ALMOND & APPLE MUESLI

Replace the raisins with ¾ cup (175 ml) chopped dried apple slices and substitute ½ cup (125 ml) of flaked almonds for the pecans. Mix the ingredients together as above.

APRICOT BRAN BREAKFAST MUFFINS

Muffins make a delicious treat for breakfast. These are very easy to make and are studded with sweet, golden apricots.

1 Soak the bran in the skim milk for 30 minutes. Meanwhile, preheat the oven to 400°F (200°C).

2 Beat the egg, molasses, oil and sugar into the soaked bran, then sift the flour, baking powder, salt and baking soda into the mixture. Add the apricots, and fold them in lightly but thoroughly, using a large spoon. If you prefer, ½ cup/125 ml of raisins can be used in place of the apricots.

3 Spoon the mixture into 8 paper-lined muffin tins and bake for 25 minutes or until they are cooked through. Serve warm.

1½ cups (375 ml) bran

⅔ cup (150 ml) skim milk

1 large egg, beaten

1 tablespoon (15 ml) molasses

3 tbsp + 1 tsp (50 ml) sunflower oil

½ cup (125 ml) light brown sugar

¾ cup (175 ml) wholewheat flour

½ teaspoon (2 ml) baking powder

Pinch each of salt and baking soda

½ cup (125 ml) dried apricots, soaked overnight, drained and finely chopped; or raisins

Makes 8

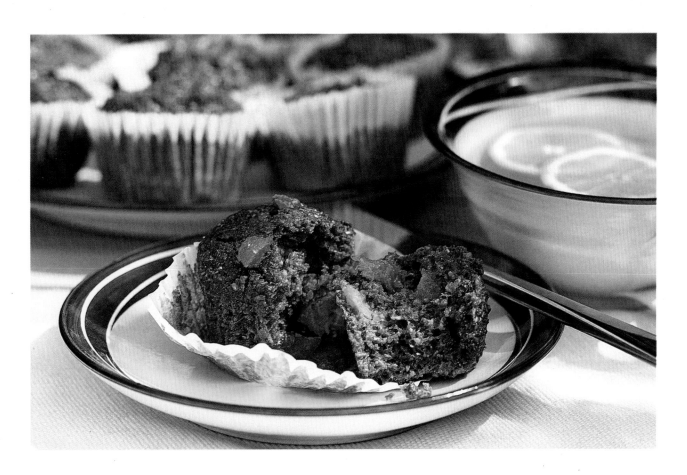

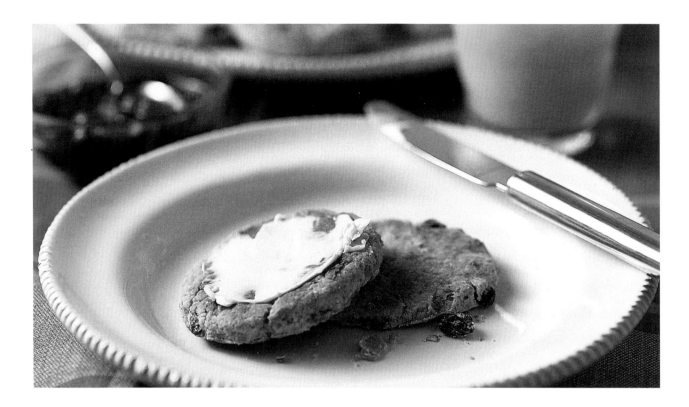

FRUITY BREAKFAST PANCAKES

½ cup (125 ml) self-rising flour

½ cup (125 ml) wholewheat flour

½ teaspoon (2 ml) baking powder

2 tablespoons (25 ml) sugar

Pinch ground cinnamon

⅓ cup (75 ml) chilled margarine

3 tablespoons (45 ml) raisins

Zest of 1 lemon, finely chopped

1 medium egg, beaten with 2 teaspoons (10 ml) skim milk

1 teaspoon (5 ml) sunflower oil

Makes 8

These breakfast pancakes are fragrant with cinnamon, lemon and juicy raisins, though you can choose any mixture of dried fruit. They are traditionally cooked on a solid cast iron griddle, but if you don't have one, use a large heavy-based frying pan.

1 Sift the flours, baking powder, sugar and cinnamon into a large bowl, adding any bran that remains in the sifter.

2 Lightly rub the margarine into the dry ingredients with your fingertips until the mixture resembles coarse breadcrumbs.

3 Stir in the raisins, add the lemon zest and fold in the egg and milk mixture, a little at a time, to make a soft dough.

4 Transfer to a lightly floured board, and roll out to about ½ inch (1 cm) thick. Cut the dough into rounds. Gather up any scraps and roll them out again until all the dough is used up.

5 Lightly grease the griddle or frying pan with half of the oil, and heat over medium heat. Place 4 pancakes on the hot surface, and cook them for 2–3 minutes on each side, until they are browned and cooked through.

6 Grease the griddle or frying pan with the rest of the oil and cook the rest of the pancakes in the same way. Serve hot, with low-fat spread, if desired.

HONEY-GRILLED GRAPEFRUIT WITH TOASTED SESAME SEEDS

Drizzled with honey, scattered with sesame seeds and grilled to perfection, your breakfast grapefruit is infused with sweet honey and nut flavors. If you don't have sesame seeds, sprinkle some toasted wheatgerm or flaked almonds on top.

1 Using a sharp kitchen knife, cut a small piece from the bottom of each grapefruit half, so that the flat base of the fruit will sit comfortably on the rack of your broiler pan.

2 Preheat the broiler. Take a grapefruit or other serrated knife and carefully cut around each grapefruit half, gently loosening the flesh from the skin. Then cut between the segments, so that they will be easy to spoon out.

3 Spoon the honey onto the top of each grapefruit half, pressing gently so that it oozes through the segments.

4 Arrange the grapefruit halves on the grill rack, and broil under a medium heat for about 2 minutes.

5 Sprinkle over the sesame seeds and broil for a further 30 seconds (no longer, or the seeds will burn). Serve immediately.

2 large pink grapefruit, halved, seeds removed

2 tablespoons (25 ml) liquid honey

2 tablespoons (25 ml) sesame seeds

Serves 4

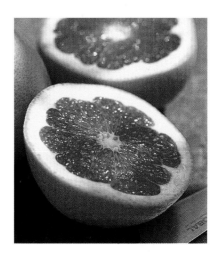

BANANA & MANGO YOGURT SMOOTHIE WITH WHEATGERM

Smoothies make a great start to your day, and taste fantastic. You can use different combinations of fruit, but make sure it is ripe.

1 Put the fruit into a blender or food processor, add the yogurt and skim milk, and process for a few seconds until smooth.

2 Pour into 2 serving glasses and chill for at least 1 hour.

3 Mix the wheatgerm and honey together, and stir the mixture into the smoothie just before serving.

1 medium banana, peeled and chopped

1 medium ripe mango, peeled and diced

1⅓ cup (325 ml) low-fat (1–2% M.F.) plain yogurt

⅔ cup (150 ml) skim milk

FOR THE TOPPING

½ cup (125 ml) wheatgerm

1 tablespoon (15 ml) liquid honey

Serves 2

PAPAYA & STRAWBERRY SMOOTHIE
Mix a chopped ripe papaya with 1 cup (250 ml) halved strawberries in a blender and then blend in the low-fat plain yogurt and skim milk as above.

SCRAMBLED EGGS WITH SMOKED SALMON

4 medium eggs

Pinch of salt and black pepper

Good pinch cayenne pepper

1 teaspoon (5 ml) sunflower oil

4 green onions, sliced

1 red bell pepper, seeded and diced

4 oz (115 g) smoked salmon, sliced

Serves 4

This creamy mixture of egg and smoked salmon is quick and easy to prepare, and the red pepper adds an interesting crunchy texture.

1 Beat the eggs with the salt, pepper and cayenne.

2 Heat the oil and stir-fry the green onions and diced peppers for a couple of minutes, until they have softened.

3 Pour the egg mixture over the onions and peppers. Stir continuously until the eggs are cooked through, but are still moist and creamy. Stir in the salmon, warm through gently and serve immediately.

EGGS FLORENTINE

4 medium eggs

1 tablespoon (15 ml) butter

1 small onion, finely chopped

6 cups (1.5 liters) leaf spinach

2 soft kaiser rolls, halved

¼ cup (50 ml) Cheddar cheese, finely grated

Salt and pepper, to taste

Serves 4

A light, balanced breakfast of poached egg on a bed of buttered spinach all piled into a kaiser roll—a perfect combination.
Remember to cook the spinach lightly so as to preserve all the natural goodness as well as a bit of bite! You can use a tablespoon (15 ml) of olive oil instead of the butter if you like.

1 Poach the eggs until they are cooked but not runny.

2 Heat the butter in a non-stick pan. Add the onion and fry for 2–3 minutes.

3 Add the spinach and stir-fry until it has just wilted and the moisture has evaporated. Season to taste.

4 Toast the halved kaiser rolls and lay them on warmed plates. Smother with the spinach and place a poached egg on top.

5 Finish with freshly ground black pepper and a little grated cheese.

SALMON KEDGEREE WITH FRESH CILANTRO

Kedgeree—sometimes called kichri—*is a dish representative of England's colonial history, traditionally made with smoked haddock, rice, boiled eggs and Indian spices. This lighter version has the delicate flavor of salmon and is highlighted with fragrant cilantro. Serve it hot on triangles of toast for a lazy weekend breakfast or Sunday brunch.*

1   Place the salmon fillets in a shallow pan with the water, wine, bay leaf, salt and pepper and bring to a boil.

2   Lower the heat and poach gently for 5 minutes. Remove from the heat and leave to cool in the cooking liquid.

3   Heat the oil in a large, heavy-based pan and gently fry the onion until softened but not browned. Stir in the curry powder and cook, stirring continuously, for a further minute. Add the rice, stir it thoroughly into the onion mixture, and set aside.

4   Once the salmon is cool enough to handle, lift it from the cooking liquid with a slotted spoon. Flake the flesh, and remove any skin and bones.

5   Strain the cooking liquid into a measuring cup, and add enough water to make 2⅓ cups (575 ml). Pour this into the rice mixture, and bring it to a boil. Stir once, lower the heat and cook for about 12–15 minutes or until the rice is tender and the liquid is absorbed.

6   Carefully fold in the salmon and eggs, trying not to break them up too much. Adjust the seasoning, if necessary, and serve hot, garnished with finely chopped fresh cilantro.

TRADITIONAL KEDGEREE

Boil the rice in vegetable stock and plenty of water, drain and set aside. Poach 10 oz (300 g) of smoked haddock in a shallow pan. Drain and flake the fish, removing any bones. Heat 1 tablespoon (15 ml) of sunflower oil and sauté 1⅓ cups (325 ml) sliced mushrooms and 1 finely chopped onion for about 5 minutes. Mix the cooked fish, rice, mushrooms and onions together. Add ⅔ cup (150 ml) of boiled peas, 1 tablespoon (15 ml) of fresh lemon or lime juice and seasoning. Place the mixture in a covered oven-proof dish and bake for 15–20 minutes at 325°F (170°C).

12 oz (350 g) salmon fillets

⅔ cup (150 ml) water

⅔ cup (150 ml) dry white wine

1 bay leaf

Salt and pepper, to taste

1 tablespoon (15 ml) sunflower oil

1 large onion, finely chopped

2 teaspoons (10 ml) curry powder

1 cup (250 ml) long-grain rice

2 medium eggs, hard-boiled and quartered

2 tablespoons (25 ml) finely chopped cilantro, to garnish

Serves 4

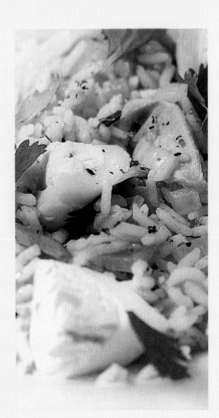

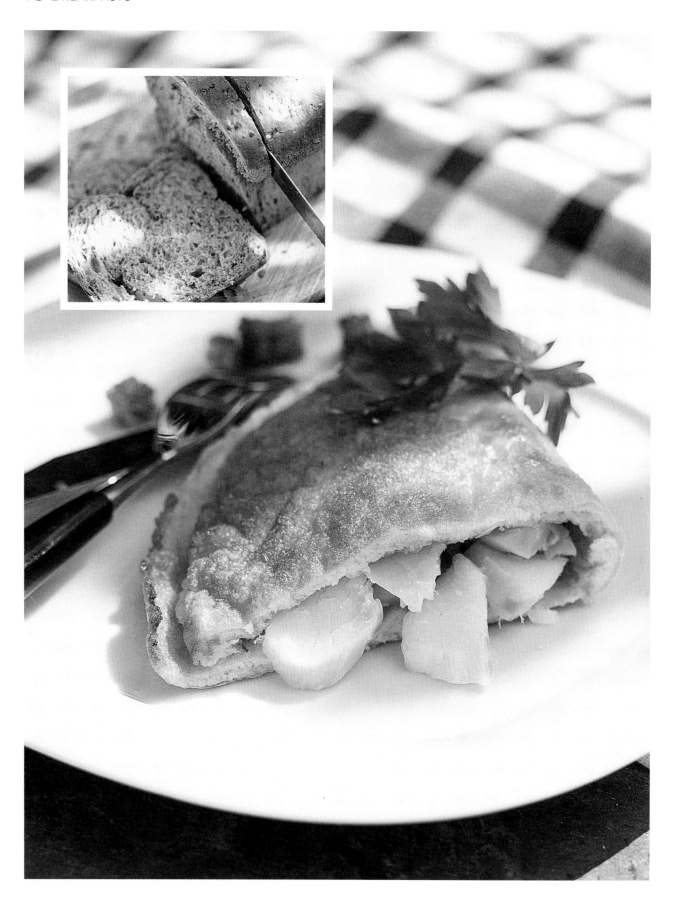

SMOKED HADDOCK SOUFFLÉ OMELET WITH CROUTONS

This feathery light, melt-in-the-mouth omelet makes a special weekend brunch for two people. If you have guests, you can simply double the quantities, use a larger omelet pan and serve four.

1 Make the croutons. Heat the oil in a large, heavy-based frying pan and fry the bread cubes on both sides until crisp. Drain on a paper towel.

2 Put the fish in a pan with enough water to cover it. Bring it to a boil, lower the heat and poach gently for 5 minutes or until cooked through. When the fish is cool enough to handle, lift it out of the cooking liquid with a slotted spoon and drain. Discard the liquid.

3 Beat the egg yolks in a large bowl and season with salt and pepper.

4 In another clean, dry, bowl, using a clean, dry, whisk, beat the whites until they stand up in soft peaks. Using a large metal spoon, fold them lightly but thoroughly into the beaten yolks.

5 Preheat the broiler to high. Meanwhile, heat the butter or margarine in an 8-inch (20-cm) non-stick omelet pan, then pour in the egg mixture.

6 Cook over a moderate heat for 4–5 minutes, gently lifting the edges of the omelet with a spatula, so that the egg mixture runs underneath and the omelet cooks through.

7 Place the pan under the grill and cook the omelet for a further 2–3 minutes until the top is set.

8 Spoon the flaked haddock over one-half of the omelet, then tilt the pan, and use a spatula to fold it in half.

9 Slide the omelet onto a warm plate and cut it in half. Scatter the top of the omelet with the croutons and serve immediately.

6 oz (175 g) smoked haddock fillet

FOR THE CROUTONS

1 tablespoon (15 ml) sunflower oil

2 medium slices wholewheat bread from a large loaf, cut into cubes

FOR THE OMELET

3 large eggs, separated

Salt and pepper, to taste

1 tablespoon (15 ml) butter or margarine

Serves 2

SUBSTITUTIONS:

If you're not used to eating fish in the morning, you can use lean peameal bacon (Canadian back bacon) as a tasty substitute for the haddock. Cook the bacon in a dry frying pan over medium heat until browned. (Use a spoonful of olive oil if needed.) Cut into bite-sized pieces and use to fill the omelet.

WILD MUSHROOM TOASTS

2¾ cups (675 ml) baby new potatoes, sliced (unpeeled)

I teaspoon (5 ml) olive oil

Salt and pepper, to taste

FOR THE MUSHROOMS

I tablespoon (15 ml) olive oil

4 medium shallots, chopped

I lb (454 g) wild mushrooms

Cooking spray

8 ripe tomatoes, halved

3 tablespoons (45 ml) chopped fresh parsley

3 tablespoons (45 ml) chopped fresh chives

2 tablespoons (25 ml) low-fat sour cream

Salt and pepper, to taste

4 slices white bread

TO SERVE

I tablespoon (15 ml) pine nuts

I tablespoon (15 ml) fresh chopped chives

Serves 4

An appetizing breakfast, that has the freshness of wild mushrooms, flavored with fresh parsley, shallots, chives and sour cream. The mushrooms are piled on top of layers of sliced potato and crusty white bread and are served with grilled tomatoes. A scattering of toasted pine nuts and chopped chives add the finishing touches.

1 Boil the potatoes until they are just cooked but still keep their shape. Drain, toss in a teaspoon (5 ml) of olive oil and season. Keep warm.

2 Heat a heavy-based frying pan and toast the pine nuts over low heat, stirring continuously. Remove the pine nuts from the heat, set them to one side and allow them to cool.

3 Meanwhile, heat the tablespoon (15 ml) of oil in a non-stick pan and fry the shallots to soften.

4 Stir in the mushrooms and fry gently for 4–5 minutes.

5 Meanwhile, spray the frying pan with cooking spray and heat. Gently place the tomatoes, skin side up, in the pan. Cook on both sides till the tomatoes are charred and soft, yet still retain their shape. Reserve until ready to use.

6 While the tomatoes are cooking, add the fresh parsley and chives to the mushrooms. Stir in the low-fat sour cream, season to taste and heat through.

7 Toast the bread lightly and place each slice onto a warmed plate. Spoon a layer of the sliced potatoes on top.

8 Pile the mushrooms onto the potatoes and top with a sprinkling of toasted pine nuts and chopped chives.

9 Add the grilled tomatoes to the plate and serve immediately while everything is hot.

POTATO CAKES

If you have any leftover mashed potatoes, transform them into a tasty treat. These pancakes can be served with lean grilled bacon and tomatoes, cold ham with grated cheese melted over the top, baked beans or a touch of butter.

1   Mash the potatoes with a little skim milk. Place all the ingredients in a large mixing bowl and mix together with your hands to make a pliable dough.

2   Take a third of the mixture, place it on a lightly floured surface and roll into a thin circle, about 6–7 inches (15–18 cm) in diameter.

3   Prick the dough all over with a fork, and cut it into 4 triangles.

4   Heat a heavy-based frying pan or griddle until very hot. Do not add any fat. Place the 4 cakes on the hot surface, and cook for about 3 minutes on each side until they are golden brown.

5   Keep the finished potato cakes warm by wrapping them in a clean dish towel and put them to one side while you make the rest. Cook the remaining 2 batches as before, and serve hot.

1⅓ cups (325 ml) mashed potato (plus skim milk as needed)

1¼ cups (300 ml) quick-cooking oats or oat bran

⅓ cup (75 ml) all-purpose flour (plus extra for dusting)

Pinch of salt

Makes 12

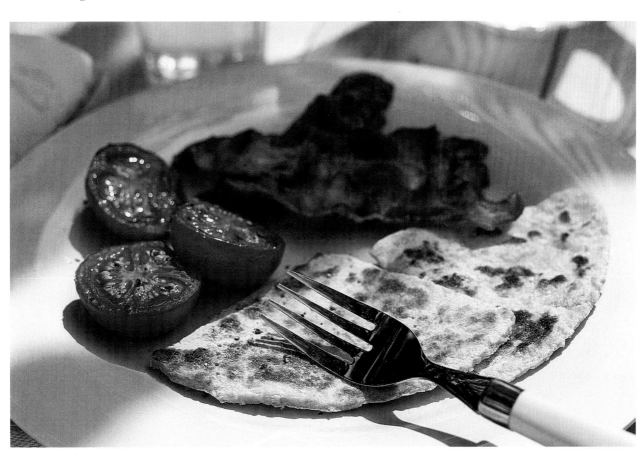

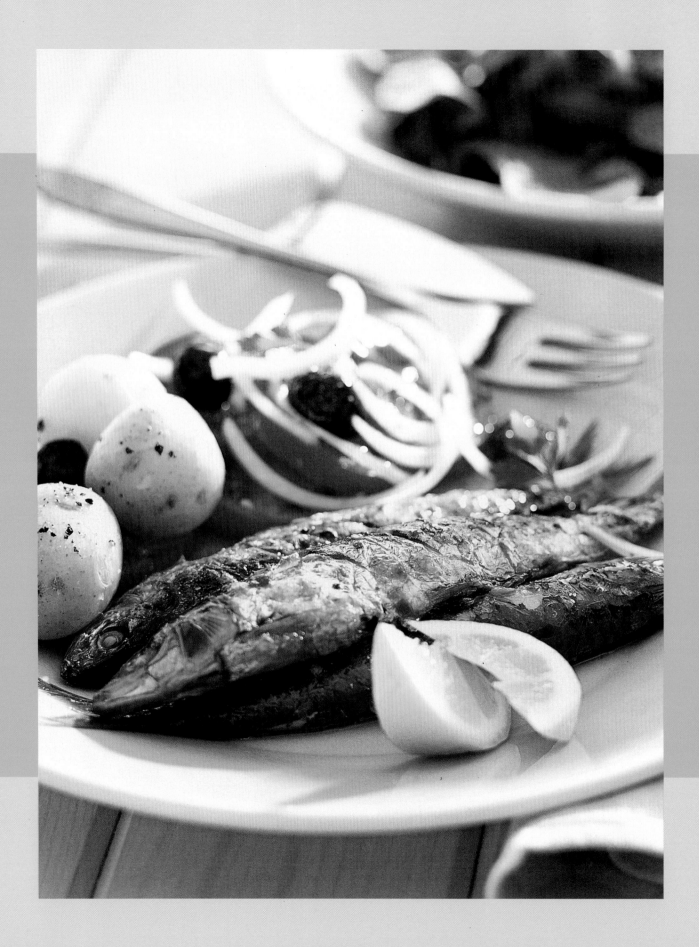

Light Meals & Snacks

2

SHRIMP & APPLE PITA POCKETS

8 oz (225 g) surimi (imitation crab), diced

3½ oz (125 ml) cooked salad shrimp

1 large apple, cored and diced

2 tablespoons (25 ml) mustard dressing

Four 4-inch (10-cm) mini pita breads

4 crisp lettuce leaves, shredded

Serves 4

Pita bread opens up into a convenient pocket that can be generously filled to make a light but satisfying meal. Try this seafood version—it's great for picnics and packed lunches.

1   In a bowl, mix the surimi, shrimp, apple and dressing together. (If you prefer, you can substitute 3½ oz (100 g) (drained weight) water-packed tuna for the shrimp.)

2   Fill the pitas with some of the lettuce and top with the seafood mix.

For mustard dressing, mix 1 teaspoon (5 ml) Dijon mustard with 2 teaspoons (10 ml) of olive oil, and 1 teaspoon (5 ml) apple cider vinegar. Add salt and pepper to taste.

LAYERED MEDITERRANEAN SANDWICH

One 12-inch (30-cm) baguette

2 teaspoons (10 ml) fat-free vinaigrette

2 medium tomatoes, sliced

2 bell peppers (one each of red and yellow), roasted, peeled, seeded and sliced

4 oz (115 g) mozzarella cheese, sliced

5 pitted black olives

Few fresh basil leaves

Salt and pepper, to taste

Serves 4

This sandwich is infused with luscious sunny, Mediterranean flavors. It also improves with keeping for up to six hours, so it's ideal to take to work or as part of a picnic lunch. You can vary the flavor of your sandwich depending on the ingredients you have available. Experiment with combinations of tuna, roasted eggplant, boiled egg slices, arugula, sliced red onions, anchovy fillets or grated carrot.

1   Cut the loaf in half horizontally and sprinkle some vinaigrette dressing over both sides of the loaf.

2   Layer the rest of the ingredients onto half of the loaf, season with salt and pepper, and sprinkle with the remainder of the vinaigrette.

3   Place the other half of the loaf on top and wrap the sandwich tightly in aluminum foil or plastic wrap.

4   Store in the refrigerator. Place a heavy object on the sandwich to help flatten it.

5   Unwrap, cut into slices and serve.

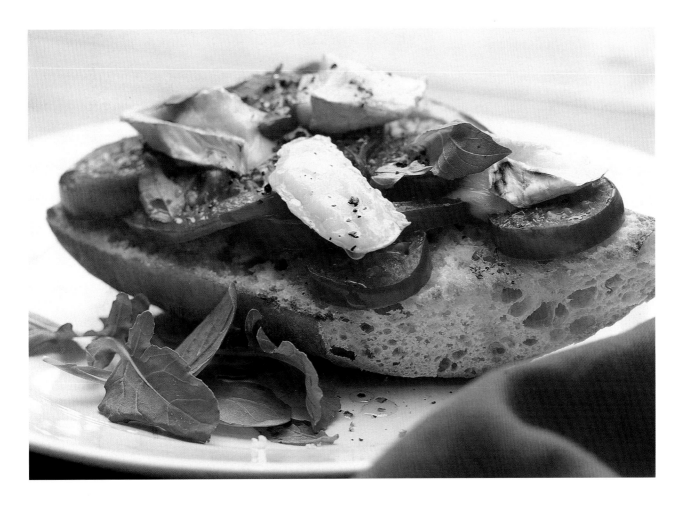

GOAT CHEESE,
TOMATO & CIABATTA GRILL

Simplicity itself, this grilled sandwich is ideal for a light lunch or supper. Use the ripest tomatoes you can find, as their sweetness will provide a delicious contrast to the sharpness of the goat cheese. It is also very good made with mozzarella cheese, using the same quantities.

1 Preheat the broiler to medium. Arrange the ciabatta slices on the broiler pan, and drizzle with the olive oil.

2 Top with the sliced tomatoes, sprinkle them with the herbs, then broil for about 3 minutes or until the tomatoes are soft and pulpy.

3 Add the cheese slices, season well, and broil for a further 3–4 minutes.

4 Serve with the mixed salad leaves, garnished with sprigs of fresh basil.

4 thick slices ciabatta or French bread, cut lengthwise

2 teaspoons (10 ml) extra virgin olive oil

4 small very ripe tomatoes, sliced

1 teaspoon (5 ml) Herbes de Provence

4 oz (115 g) goat cheese, thinly sliced

Salt and pepper, to taste

1 cup (250 ml) mixed salad greens, to serve

4 small sprigs fresh basil, to garnish

Serves 2

PORTUGUESE SARDINE SALAD

Fresh sardines are absolutely delicious, although not always available. Alternatively, buy them frozen. The traditional Portuguese way of serving them is with plain boiled potatoes and a simple salad of tomatoes, onion and black olives.

2¼ lbs (1 kg) fresh, cleaned Portuguese sardines (thawed if frozen)

Pinch coarse sea salt

1 tablespoon (15 ml) lemon juice

1 teaspoon (5 ml) piri-piri or other hot pepper sauce

1½ lbs (700 g) new potatoes in their skins (about 11 medium)

FOR THE SALAD

6 medium tomatoes, sliced

1 small onion, thinly sliced

⅓ cup (75 ml) black olives

2 tablespoons (25 ml) olive oil

2 teaspoons (10 ml) white wine vinegar

Salt and pepper, to taste

Serves 6

1 Preheat the broiler to high. Make 2 or 3 slits in the plumpest part of each sardine using a sharp knife.

2 Mix together the sea salt, lemon juice and hot sauce and rub into the slits.

3 Cook the sardines under a hot broiler for 5–8 minutes each side—the grilling time will depend on their size.

4 While the sardines are cooking, boil and drain the potatoes.

5 Make the salad. Put the tomatoes, onion slices and olives in a bowl. To make the dressing, put the olive oil, wine vinegar and seasoning in a screw top jar, and shake thoroughly.

6 Serve the sardines with the potatoes, and the salad tossed in the dressing on the side.

TUNA & DILL DIP WITH VEGETABLE CRUDITÉS

These juicy, crunchy vegetable sticks make a piquant and colorful contrast to the tuna dip, which is scented with the delicious aniseed flavor of fresh dill. A perfect summer snack.

7 oz (220 g) canned tuna in water, drained

4 tablespoons (50 ml) fat-free vinaigrette dressing

½ cup (125 ml) low-fat (1–2% M.F.) plain yogurt

½ cup (125 ml) fresh dill, finely chopped

Salt and pepper, to taste

1 large seedless cucumber, cut into strips

3 medium carrots, peeled, cut into sticks

3 stalks celery, cut into 3-inch (8-cm) pieces

2 red bell peppers, seeded, cut into strips

Serves 4

1 Prepare the tuna dip by mixing together the tuna, vinaigrette dressing, low-fat yogurt, dill and seasonings. Chill the mixture.

2 When ready to serve, place the tuna in the center of a chilled plate. Surround with the crudités and serve.

AVOCADO WITH CHICKEN & WALNUT SALAD

Here's something special—a light but luscious meal that will gratify your tastebuds. The flavors of the avocados and walnuts combine perfectly with the chicken, and this is ideal for lunch or supper.

1   Put the avocado slices into a bowl with the lemon juice and mix gently to coat. Set to one side.

2   Heat the olive oil in a wok or non-stick frying pan, and stir-fry the chicken strips for 3–4 minutes or until they are cooked through.

3   Add the pimiento slices and stir-fry for 1 further minute.

4   Remove from the heat, then drain the lemon juice from the avocados, and stir it into the chicken. Mix in the seasonings, mustard and sugar.

5   Arrange the avocado slices onto 4 serving plates, add the chicken salad and serve garnished with the walnuts.

---

4 avocados, peeled, pitted and sliced

2 tablespoons (25 ml) lemon juice

FOR THE SALAD

2 tablespoons (25 ml) extra virgin olive oil

3 x 5 oz (150 g) skinless, boneless chicken breasts, cut into thin strips

½ cup (125 ml) canned red pimiento, drained and finely sliced

Salt and pepper, to taste

2 teaspoons (10 ml) Dijon mustard

1 teaspoon (5 ml) sugar

½ cup (125 ml) chopped walnuts, to garnish

Serves 4

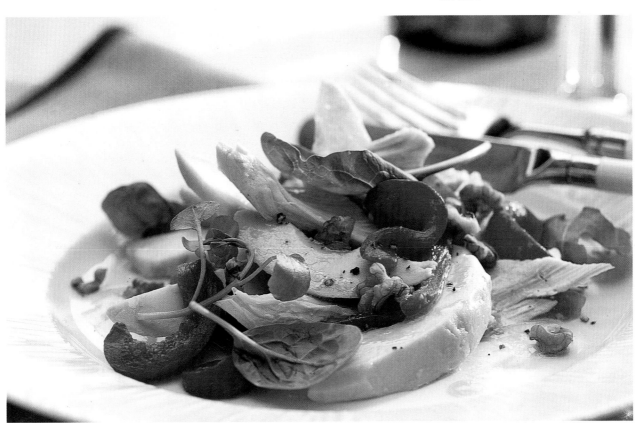

WARM LENTILS & KIDNEY BEANS WITH BACON

1⅓ cups (325 ml) uncooked Puy or green lentils

1¼ cups (300 ml) canned red kidney beans, drained and rinsed

Salt and pepper, to taste

½ teaspoon (2 ml) hot pepper sauce (or to taste)

1 tablespoon (15 ml) olive oil

1 medium onion, finely chopped

6 oz (175 g) lean, smoked bacon, diced

¼ cup (50 ml) low-fat sour cream and a sprinkling of paprika, to garnish

Serves 4

This is best made with green Puy lentils—they're available from large supermarkets or specialty food shops. However, if you can't get them, use any lentils, and follow the package instructions for cooking times. This is a great dish for people with diabetes, as the beans and lentils allow blood glucose levels to rise slowly.

1 Cook the lentils according to the package instructions—if you are using Puy lentils, this should take about 35 minutes. Drain the lentils.

2 Place the cooked, drained lentils in a bowl, and add the drained kidney beans, seasonings and hot pepper sauce. Mix together thoroughly.

3 Heat the oil in a non-stick heavy-based frying pan, and gently sauté the onion for 2–3 minutes until softened but not browned.

4 Add the bacon and cook, stirring, for a further 3 minutes or until bacon is cooked and crisp.

5 Add the bacon and onions to the lentil and bean mixture, mix thoroughly and serve garnished with low-fat sour cream and a sprinkling of paprika.

SWEET POTATO & VEGETABLE STEW

1 tablespoon (15 ml) olive oil

2 garlic cloves, crushed

1 medium onion, chopped

1 green bell pepper, seeded and diced

2¼ cups (550 ml) sweet potatoes (about 2 medium), peeled and chopped into cubes

4 large tomatoes, chopped

1 teaspoon (5 ml) Herbes de Provence

Salt and pepper, to taste

2¼ cups (550 ml) fresh or frozen whole green beans, thawed

2¼ cups (550 ml) canned red kidney beans, drained and rinsed

3 tablespoons (45 ml) freshly chopped parsley

Serves 4

A warming stew of fresh vegetables with a mix of green beans and red kidney beans. The sweet potato makes this into a delightfully unusual dish.

1 Heat the oil in a large pan with a lid. Fry the garlic, onion and green pepper until they have softened.

2 Add the sweet potato, tomatoes, herbs and seasonings. Stir well, cover and cook for 20–25 minutes until the sweet potato is cooked but not mushy.

3 Add the green beans and the kidney beans to the potato stew, stir and allow to cook until the green beans are done.

4 When cooked, adjust the seasonings and serve hot, topped with parsley.

TUSCAN BREAD SALAD WITH RED ONION & MOZZARELLA

This is a variation of a traditional Italian peasant snack, and is an ideal way of using up stale bread. It has to be the right kind of bread, though—a coarse, dense-textured loaf is just what you need. Ciabatta is a good choice, and it should be at least 3 or 4 days old.

1 Sprinkle the bread on both sides with just enough water to moisten it.

2 Place the slices on individual serving plates and sprinkle the wine vinegar over one side only. Season with salt and pepper.

3 Arrange layers of vegetables and cheese on each slice of bread, drizzle with the olive oil, and serve garnished with sprigs of fresh basil.

4 thick slices stale ciabatta or French bread, cut lengthwise

2 tablespoons (25 ml) red wine vinegar

Salt and pepper, to taste

6 medium ripe tomatoes, sliced

2 small red onions, thinly sliced

1 stalk celery, including leaves, thinly sliced

6 oz (175 g) mozzarella cheese, thinly sliced

3 tablespoons (45 ml) extra virgin olive oil

4 small sprigs basil, to garnish

Serves 4

HOMEMADE POPCORN

Popcorn is a healthy snack that won't send your blood glucose soaring. It is packed with slowly absorbed fiber and by making it yourself, you can make sure it's low in fat.

1 Heat a heavy-based non-stick pan with a tight-fitting lid over high heat until it is very hot. Carefully pour in the oil and keep the heat turned up high.

2 Add the corn, then cover with the lid. Shake the pan over the heat. The corn will start to pop and bounce off the lid. Remove the pan from the heat immediately after the popping stops.

3 Season with a little salt and as much lemon juice as you like, and serve.

1 teaspoon (5 ml) corn oil

2 heaping tablespoons (30–40 ml) popping corn

Pinch salt

Fresh lemon juice, to taste

Serves 2

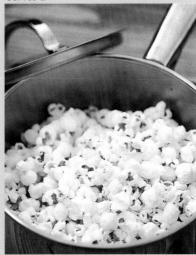

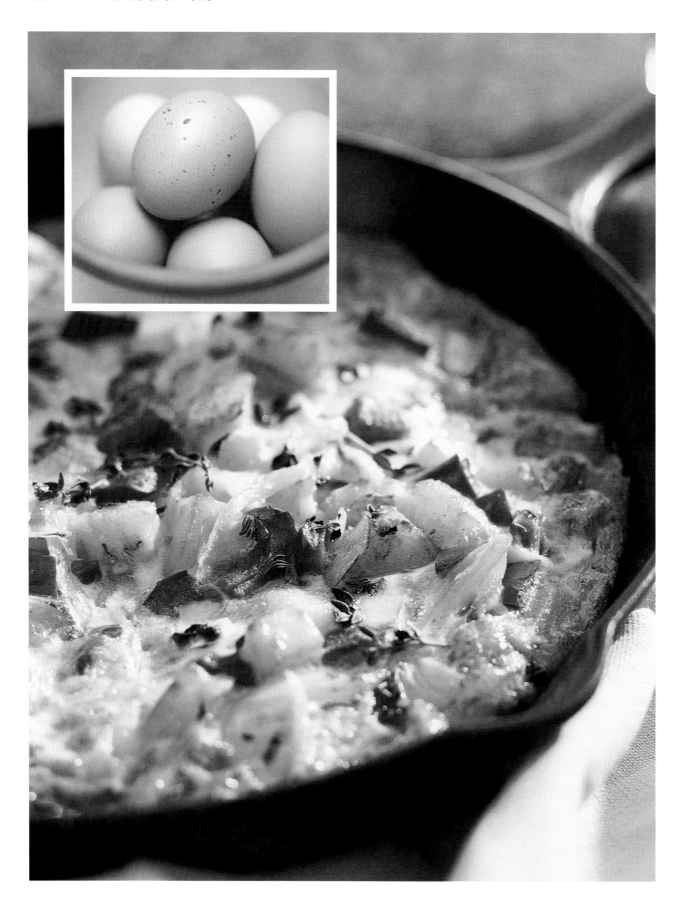

POTATO, RED PEPPER & ONION FRITTATA

This typical Italian-style omelet is flavored with tasty onion and peppers. It is delicious served hot, warm or cold and makes a great picnic dish.

About 4 medium-sized potatoes, peeled and diced

1 tablespoon (15 ml) olive oil

1 medium onion, peeled and thinly sliced

1 red bell pepper, seeded and diced

4 large eggs

1 tablespoon (15 ml) cold water

Salt and pepper, to taste

1 teaspoon (5 ml) chopped fresh thyme or oregano

Serves 4

1 Preheat the broiler to high. Boil the diced potatoes in lightly salted water for 5 minutes or until they are just tender. Drain them well.

2 Heat the oil in a large, heavy-based, non-stick frying pan and gently sauté the onion for 3–4 minutes until it is softened but not browned.

3 Add the cooked potato and red pepper, increase the heat slightly and cook for a further 2–3 minutes, stirring gently, until the potatoes turn golden.

4 Beat the eggs with the cold water, season to taste, then mix in the herbs.

5 Pour the eggs evenly over the vegetables in the pan and cook over medium heat for 2–3 minutes until the base is nicely browned.

6 Transfer the pan to the broiler and cook for a further 2 minutes or until the top is set and a deep golden brown. Serve in wedges.

VEGETABLE GRATIN

Fast and tasty, this can be served as an accompaniment or as a light meal with warm crusty French bread.

3 medium carrots, peeled and sliced

1 medium cauliflower, trimmed and divided into florets

½ head of broccoli, trimmed and divided into florets

¾ cup (175 ml) frozen small peas

⅓ cup (75 ml) package instant cheese sauce mix (or 3 tablespoons (45 ml) prepared cheese sauce)

1 teaspoon (5 ml) Dijon mustard

Salt and coarsely ground pepper

2 tablespoons (25 ml) finely grated Cheddar cheese

2 ripe tomatoes, sliced lengthwise

Serves 4

1 Cook the carrots in a little boiling water for about 3 minutes.

2 Add the cauliflower, broccoli and peas, cover and cook until the vegetables are just tender. Drain and put the vegetables in a large, lightly greased flameproof dish, cover and keep warm.

3 Make up the cheese sauce as directed on the package. Stir in the mustard and the seasoning. Preheat the broiler to medium.

4 Pour the sauce over the vegetables and mix gently. Top with the grated cheese and tomato slices.

5 Broil under medium heat for 5 minutes. Serve immediately.

PIZZA WITH TRI-COLORED PEPPERS & BEANS

FOR THE BASE

1 cup (250 ml) all-purpose white flour

1 cup (250 ml) wholewheat flour

1 teaspoon (5 ml) dry yeast

¼ teaspoon (2 ml) salt

⅔ cup (150 ml) lukewarm water

1 tablespoon (15 ml) sunflower oil

FOR THE TOPPING

2 teaspoons (10 ml) olive oil

1 medium red onion, roughly chopped

1 red bell pepper, seeded and sliced

1 yellow bell pepper, seeded and sliced

1 green bell pepper, seeded and sliced

2¼ cups (550 ml) canned red kidney beans, rinsed and drained

Salt and pepper, to taste

2 tablespoons (25 ml) tomato paste

1½ cups (375 ml) canned chopped tomatoes, seasoned with herbs with garlic

4 oz (115 g) mozzarella cheese, grated

½ cup (125 ml) fresh basil leaves, torn

Serves 4

This is a gloriously colorful pizza, and has lots of slowly absorbed fiber to keep your blood glucose steady. You could buy the base ready-made, of course, and just use the topping. However, it's much nicer to prepare your own – then you'll know how pizza really should taste.

1 Preheat the oven to 425°F (220°C). Sift the white and wholewheat flours into a large bowl, then stir in the yeast and salt.

2 Make a well in the center of the flour mixture, and gradually mix in the lukewarm water and oil to form a soft dough.

3 Transfer the dough to a lightly floured board, and knead it for about 10 minutes until it is smooth and elastic.

4 Return the dough to the bowl (cleaned, if necessary), cover with a dish towel and leave it to stand in a warm place for about 1 hour or until the dough has doubled in size.

5 While the dough is rising, heat the oil for the topping in a heavy-based non-stick pan, and stir-fry the onion and peppers for 3 minutes until they are soft but not browned.

6 Add the kidney beans and season to taste. Remove the pan from the heat and put it aside.

7 Roll out the risen dough into a large circle, about 15–18 inches (38–45 cm) in diameter. Place it on a large, oiled, baking sheet or pizza pan.

8 Cover the pizza base with tomato paste, then spread with the chopped tomatoes. Top with the cooked vegetables, then sprinkle with the grated mozzarella and basil leaves.

9 Bake near the top of the oven for 25–30 minutes until the cheese is golden and bubbling. Serve immediately.

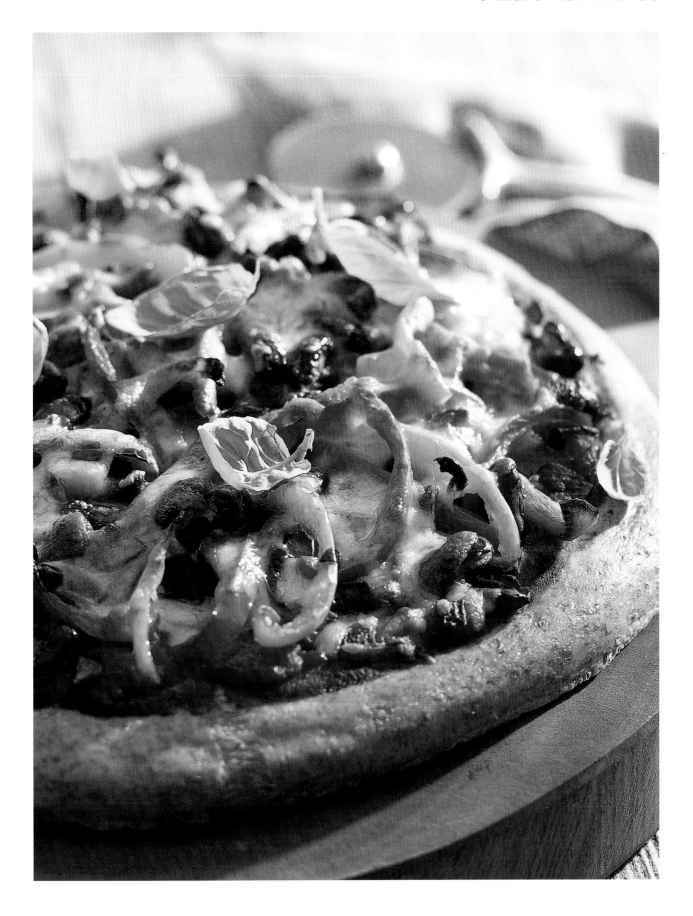

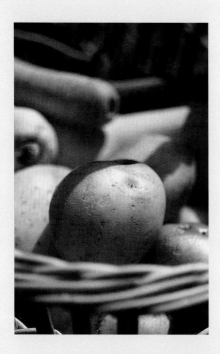

4 large baking potatoes

1 tablespoon (15 ml) sunflower oil

Serves 4

STUFFED BAKED POTATOES

Baked potatoes are cozy and comforting—a true family favorite. They're also a boon to those with diabetes—the starchy carbohydrate they contain, coupled with fiber in the skin, makes them especially nutritious. Traditional oven-baked potatoes are unbeatable, and you can be inventive with the filling of your choice.

1 Preheat the oven to 400°F (200°C).

2 Scrub the potatoes well and, while they are still damp, prick them in several places with a fork. Then rub them all over with the oil.

3 Bake the potatoes in the center of the oven for about 1 hour 15 minutes, or until the skins are nice and crisp and the centers are cooked through.

4 Remove the potatoes from the oven. When they are cool enough to handle, cut them in half lengthwise, and carefully scoop out most of the flesh into a bowl, leaving the skins intact.

5 Mix the cooked potato with your choice of the following fillings, and proceed as instructed for each filling method.

AVOCADO WITH SHRIMP
Scoop out the flesh of a large, ripe avocado into a bowl, and beat in 1 tablespoon (15 ml) low-fat sour cream. Stir in ½ teaspoon (2 ml) hot pepper sauce and 3½ oz (100 g) cooked, peeled shrimp. Mix together with the cooked potato flesh, pile the mixture back into the potato shells, and return to the oven for 5 minutes before serving.

TUNA TRICOLOR
Mix 4 oz (115 g) (drained weight) tuna packed in water with the cooked potato, season to taste and spoon into the potato shells. Return the potatoes to the oven and reheat for 5 minutes. Meanwhile, prepare the topping. Mix together ¼ cup (50 ml) each of diced red and green bell pepper and ¼ cup (50 ml) corn kernels with 2 tablespoons (25 ml) reduced-calorie mayonnaise. Pile on top of the potatoes before serving.

SMOKED HAM WITH PESTO SAUCE
Make half the quantity of pesto sauce (see page 52) and stir into the bowl of cooked potato. Add 3½ oz (100 g) diced lean smoked ham and mix thoroughly. Pile the mixture back into the potato shells and top with 2 tablespoons (25 ml) Parmesan cheese shavings. (Use a potato peeler.) Return to the oven for 5 minutes before serving.

BAKED CHEESY TRIANGLES

A quick grilled cheese can be made quite memorable with a few tasty additions. Serve these with a simple lettuce and cherry tomato salad or with the baked tomato and olive salad on page 81.

1 Preheat the oven to 350°F (180°C).

2 Cover 4 of the slices of bread with the cheese and the parsley, then place the remaining slices of bread on top.

3 Cut each sandwich into 4 triangles and place in a shallow, lightly greased ovenproof dish.

4 Whisk the egg and the milk together with the herbs and pepper.

5 Pour the egg and herb mixture over the sandwiches and bake in the oven for 15 minutes until golden brown.

8 slices bread, with crusts removed

1 cup (250 ml) low-fat Cheddar cheese, grated

2 tablespoons (25 ml) freshly chopped parsley

1 medium egg, beaten

⅔ cup (150 ml) low-fat milk

Good pinch of Herbes de Provence

Coarse black pepper

Serves 4

STUFFED PEPPERS

The traditional recipe for stuffed peppers can take around 40 minutes in the oven, not including preparation time for the rice filling. This method takes a less conventional but easy shortcut. The peppers cook in boiling water while you prepare the filling, so no time is wasted. Use this recipe for leftovers too. Serve with red cabbage coleslaw (see page 83) and bread.

1 Cut a circle around the stem end of each pepper and remove the seeds. Put this circle back onto the peppers to form a lid. Place the peppers upright in a saucepan half-filled with boiling water. Return to a boil, cover and cook for 5–8 minutes to soften.

2 Meanwhile, heat the oil in a non-stick pan. Add the onion and garlic and fry over gentle heat until the onion is softened.

3 Add the peas, corn and seasonings to the pan with a few tablespoons (20–30 ml) of hot water. Cover with a tight-fitting lid and cook the vegetables over high heat for a few minutes.

4 Add the parsley and cooked rice to the vegetables and stir gently.

5 Spoon the rice mixture into the peppers, sprinkle with grated cheese and cover with the pepper "lids." Serve hot.

4 red bell peppers

2 teaspoons (10 ml) corn oil

1 medium onion, finely chopped

2 cloves garlic, crushed

1 cup (250 ml) frozen peas

1 cup (250 ml) frozen corn

1 teaspoon (5 ml) Herbes de Provence

Salt and black pepper

2 tablespoons (25 ml) fresh parsley, chopped

1⅓ cup (325 ml) cooked long grain rice

⅓ cup (75 ml) reduced-fat Cheddar cheese, grated

Serves 4

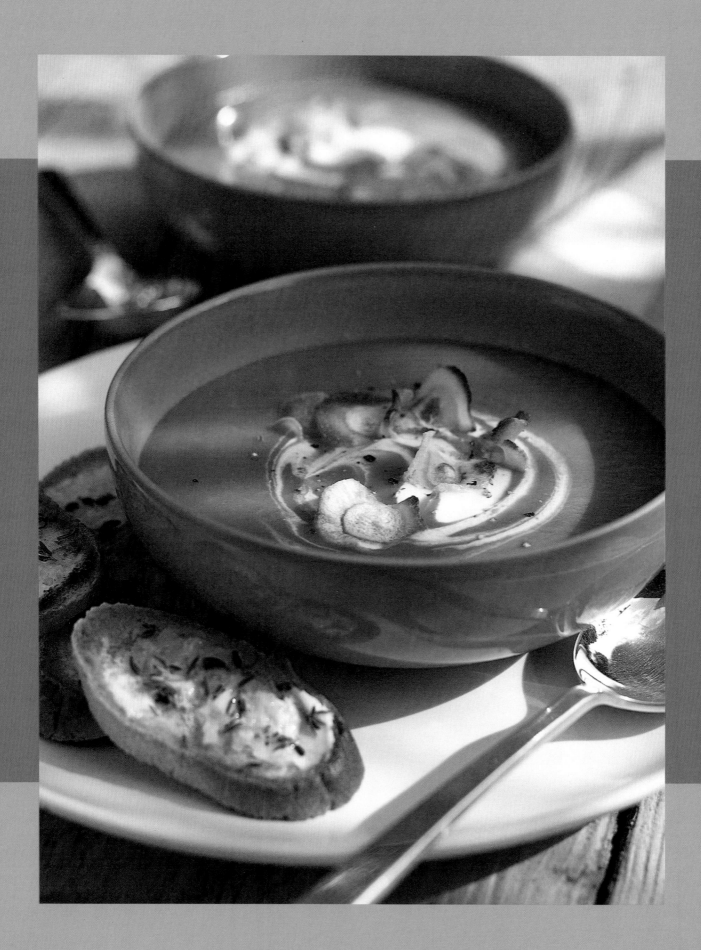

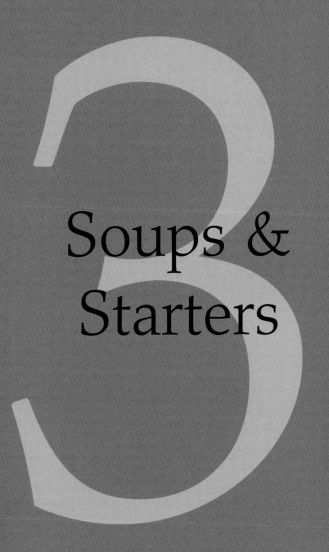

Soups & Starters

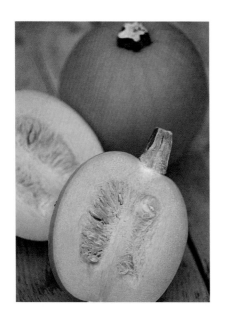

PUMPKIN SOUP WITH ROAST PARSNIP CHIPS

The golden flesh of pumpkin makes a creamy, appetizing soup bursting with enticing garlic and ginger aromas. This is delicious with hot garlic bread on a chilly day.

1. Preheat the oven to 400°F (200°C). Cut the pumpkin into 2-inch (5 cm) chunks, and put them into an ovenproof dish with the ginger. Roast in the oven for 20 minutes. (If using canned pumpkin, proceed to the next step and roast the ginger along with the parsnip.)

2. Meanwhile prepare the chips. Using a pastry brush, coat the slices of parsnip with corn oil, and lay them on an baking tray.

3. Roast the parsnip slices for 20 minutes in the oven, until they are crisp and golden, then set aside.

4. Make the soup. In a large pan, heat the oil and gently cook the onion and crushed garlic until soft.

5. Add the roasted (or canned) pumpkin and ginger and pour in the vegetable stock. Bring to the boil and simmer gently for 15 minutes until the pumpkin and vegetables are tender.

6. Pour the mixture into a blender and purée for about 1–2 minutes until it is smooth and creamy. Return the soup to the pan, and bring it back to the boil. Stir in the yogurt and adjust the seasoning.

7. Ladle into heated bowls and sprinkle with the parsnip chips for garnish.

FOR THE SOUP

2½ lbs (1 kg) pumpkin (about ¾ lb (375 g) flesh, peeled and seeded) or 3 cups (750 ml) canned pumpkin

2½ tablespoons (37 ml) ginger root, peeled and sliced

2 teaspoons (10 ml) corn oil

1 medium onion, peeled and finely chopped

2 cloves garlic, peeled and crushed

3 cups (750 ml) vegetable stock

1 cup (250 ml) low-fat (1–2% M.F.) yogurt

FOR THE CHIPS

3 medium parsnips, peeled and finely sliced

2 teaspoons (10 ml) corn oil

Serves 4–6

SWEET POTATO SOUP WITH CASSAVA CHIPS
Use 2½ lbs (1 kg) of chopped sweet potato and roast with a stick of cinnamon and a bay leaf. Follow the rest of the recipe as above. To make the chips, finely slice 7 oz (200 g) fresh peeled cassava root and roast until crisp and browned.

BEAN & PASTA SOUP WITH BASIL

This is a deeply satisfying, rustic, Italian-style soup, packed full of hearty vegetables, beans and pasta. It makes a tasty, wholesome lunch served with warm, crusty bread.

1 Drain the tomatoes, setting aside the juice for later.

2 In a large pan, heat the oil and cook the onion until soft. Add the stock, reduce the heat to low, cover and simmer for 5 minutes.

3 Add the green beans, zucchini and the reserved tomato juice. Season to taste, then simmer for 30 minutes.

4 Stir in the vermicelli and navy beans. Simmer for a further 10 minutes.

5 Mix the pesto and tomatoes together and add to the soup. Return to a boil, then serve immediately, sprinkled with the basil leaves.

½ cup (125 ml) canned peeled tomatoes

1 tablespoon (15 ml) olive oil

1 medium onion, thinly sliced

4 cups (1 liter) chicken stock

1 cup (250 ml) fresh green beans, cut into ½ inch (1 cm) lengths

2 small zucchini, diced

Salt and pepper, to taste

2 oz (60 g) vermicelli

1¼ cups (300 ml) canned navy beans, drained and rinsed

½ cup (125 ml) pesto sauce

Few fresh basil leaves, to garnish

Serves 4–6

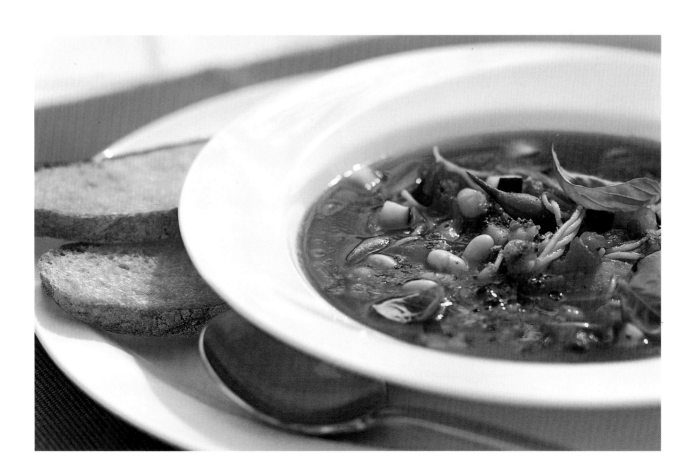

RED LENTIL SOUP

This classic dish is a perfect marriage of earthy lentils with fragrant ham. Lentils are highly effective at slowing down the rise in your blood glucose, so they are an excellent choice for people with diabetes.

1 medium ham hock

4 cups (1 liter) water

2½ cups (625 ml) rutabaga, peeled and cut into small chunks

2 medium carrots, peeled and grated

1⅓ cups (325 ml) red lentils, washed

Serves 4–6

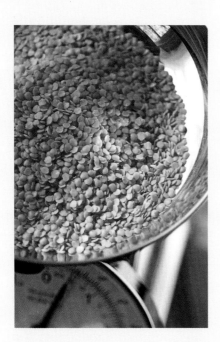

1   In a large soup pot, cover the ham hock with the water and boil for 1 hour.

2   Add the rutabaga, carrots and lentils and simmer for 30 minutes. Remove the ham pieces and the rutabaga, and either keep them warm to eat as a main course, or put them in the refrigerator to use for another meal.

3   Let the soup cool slightly, then pour it into a blender and purée for about 1 minute, adding some more water if it is too thick.

4   Reheat thoroughly before serving.

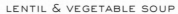

LENTIL & VEGETABLE SOUP
Omit the ham and water and substitute a good quality vegetable stock instead. This will shorten the preparation and cooking time to only 45 minutes. Use 1 cup (250 ml) red lentils and simmer them with 2 stalks of chopped celery, ¾ cup (175 ml) peeled, chopped potato and the other vegetables as above. Garnish with a swirl of low-fat plain yogurt and a sprinkle of curry powder.

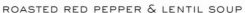

ROASTED RED PEPPER & LENTIL SOUP
Roast 2 red bell peppers under a preheated broiler until they become slightly charred. Seed and chop the peppers and add to the rutabaga and lentil mixture. Continue as above.

SPINACH & ONION SOUP

There is something satisfying about homemade soup! This recipe makes an ideal starter for any dinner party.

1 tablespoon (15 ml) vegetable oil

2 medium onions, thinly sliced

3¾ cups (900 ml) vegetable stock

1 bay leaf

Salt and pepper

⅔ cup (150 ml) white wine

6 cups (1.5 liters) leaf spinach

Serves 4

1   Heat the oil in a saucepan and fry the onions for about 5–8 minutes over low heat, until they have softened.

2   Pour in the stock and bring to a boil. Add the bay leaf and the seasonings. Cover and simmer for 10 minutes.

3   Pour in the wine and add the spinach. Continue to cook, but only until the spinach has wilted slightly.

4   Remove the bay leaf and serve hot.

FISH & POTATO SOUP

This is a delicately flavored soup, suffused with lovely smoky aromas from the fish. Be careful that you don't overcook it—the fish and potatoes should have a slightly firm texture. Cod is a suitable alternative to haddock.

1 Put the the haddock in a large saucepan, add the water and cook over a low heat for 15 minutes.

2 Remove the fish from the water, flake it roughly and set it aside.

3 Add the onions, white pepper and potatoes to the remaining stock, then cover and cook over medium heat for 20 minutes.

4 Remove the pan from the heat, mash the potatoes in the pan, leaving a few chunky pieces for texture. Return the pan to low heat, pour in the milk and add the flaked fish.

5 Simmer for 1 minute (being careful not to boil), season with the salt (if needed) and serve immediately, sprinkled with the chopped parsley.

1 lb (454 g) smoked haddock
1¼ cups (300 ml) water
2 large onions, finely chopped
½ teaspoon (2 ml) white pepper
1 lb (454 g) potatoes, peeled and sliced (makes about 3 cups/750 ml)
1¾ cups (425 ml) low-fat milk
Pinch of salt
2 tablespoons (25 ml) finely chopped parsley, to garnish
Serves 4–6

SHRIMP CHOWDER
Use only ½ lb (225 g) smoked haddock and add 1½ cups (375 ml) corn to the onions and potatoes and cook as above. After mashing the potatoes, return the mixture to the pan with ½ lb (225 g) cooked peeled shrimp.

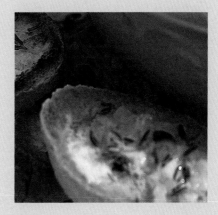

GARLIC BREAD

Commercially made garlic bread is often high in fat, but this easy version will help you to keep your weight on an even keel. It makes a wonderfully fragrant accompaniment to homemade soups

1 Preheat the broiler to medium. Cut the French bread into 8 diagonal slices, place them under the broiler and toast the slices on one side.

2 Mix the margarine, garlic and thyme together. Spread the garlic mixture evenly over the untoasted side of the bread slices.

3 Arrange the slices of bread on the broiler pans, flavored side up, and broil until lightly browned. Serve immediately.

8-inch (20 cm) loaf of French bread
⅓ cup (75 ml) reduced-calorie margarine
1 clove garlic, crushed, or 1 teaspoon (5 ml) ready-made garlic purée
1 teaspoon (5 ml) finely chopped fresh thyme
Serves 4

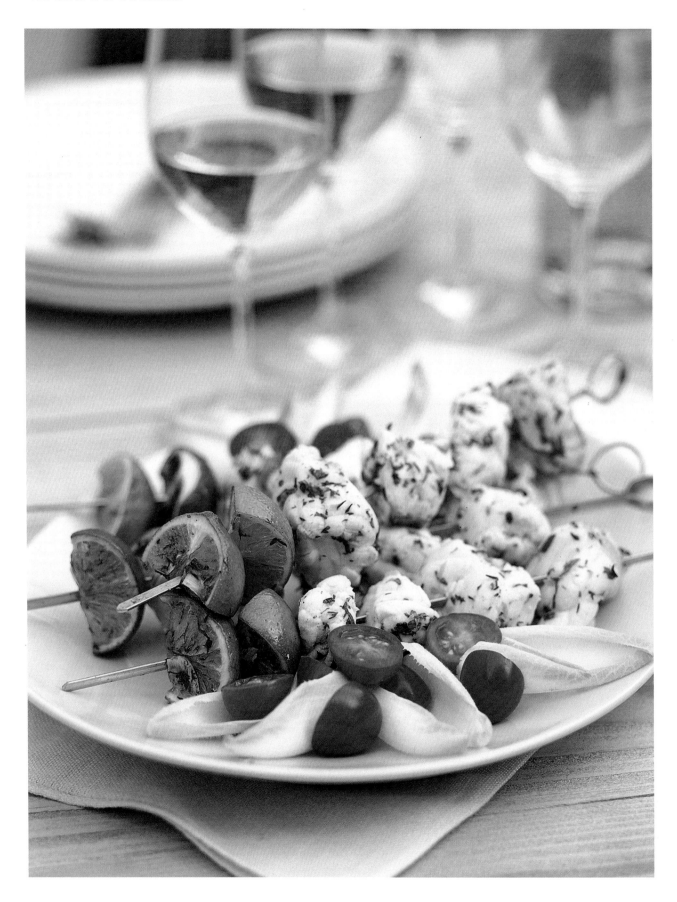

GARLIC TIGER SHRIMP

Tiger shrimp are ideal for this dish as they are firm, plump, and full of briny juices. Serve them sizzling hot, and have plenty of crusty bread on hand to soak up the garlic-scented sauce.

1 Preheat the oven to 400°F (200°C). Put the olive oil and garlic in a large, shallow ovenproof dish and heat in the oven for 2–3 minutes. You need to watch carefully so that the garlic does not start to brown.

2 Add the shrimp, and turn them in the hot oil until they are completely coated. Return them to the oven and bake for a further 3 minutes until they are pink and cooked through.

3 Serve immediately, sprinkled with freshly chopped parsley. Serve accompanied by lemon wedges for squeezing.

1 tablespoon (15 ml) olive oil

2 cloves garlic, peeled and thinly sliced

½ lb (225 g) large raw shrimp (such as tiger shrimp), peeled

Freshly chopped parsley and 1 lemon, cut into 4 wedges, to garnish

Serves 4

BAKED SEAFOOD
Defrost ½ lb (225 g) cooked seafood cocktail and use this instead of the shrimp. Add a handful of freshly chopped chives with the parsley.

MONKFISH KABOBS WITH LEMON & THYME

Monkfish has a fine flavor, and is ideal for kabobs as it keeps its nice, firm texture. If it's not available, use cod, haddock or another firm fish. Serve with warm crusty bread and a crisp green salad.

1 Preheat the broiler to medium, and line the broiler pan with aluminum foil.

2 Cut the fish fillets into chunks and place them in a bowl. Stir in the olive oil, garlic, lemon zest and juice, thyme, cilantro and seasoning.

3 Thread the fish pieces onto 4 skewers. Secure the ends with lime wedges.

4 Grill, turning occasionally, for about 5–8 minutes. It is important to make sure that the fish does not overcook.

1 lb, 7 oz (650 g) monkfish fillet

1 tablespoon (15 ml) olive oil

2 cloves garlic, crushed

Zest and juice of 1 lemon

2 tablespoons (25 ml) freshly chopped thyme

2 tablespoons (25 ml) freshly chopped cilantro

Salt and pepper, to taste

2 limes, quartered

Serves 4

HONEY-GLAZED CHICKEN WINGS

12 chicken wings

1 inch (2½ cm) ginger root, crushed

2 cloves garlic, crushed

1 teaspoon (5 ml) chili powder

2 teaspoons (10 ml) liquid honey

2 teaspoons (10 ml) coarse-grain mustard

1 teaspoon (5 ml) cider vinegar

2 tablespoons (25 ml) white wine vinegar

Salt and pepper, to taste

Serves 4

Chicken wings make a delicious appetizer, and this recipe transforms them into irresistibly tasty morsels.

1 Preheat the broiler to medium. Line a large flameproof dish with aluminum foil.

2 Put the chicken wings into a bowl, add the remaining ingredients, and mix together thoroughly.

3 Arrange the coated wings in the dish, making sure that they don't overlap.

4 Cook under the broiler for about 20 minutes, turning once or twice during cooking. Serve the wings hot or cold.

SAUTÉED CHICKEN LIVERS WITH FENNEL

2 teaspoons (10 ml) corn oil

1 medium fennel bulb, sliced

Salt and pepper

1 teaspoon (5 ml) all-purpose flour

½ lb (225 g) chicken livers

3 tablespoons (45 ml) chopped parsley

1 tablespoon (15 ml) red wine vinegar

Serves 4

Chicken livers have a delicate taste compared to other organ meats. Liver is an excellent source of iron, vitamin B12 and protein, but make sure you don't overcook it as it can then become tough. The fennel adds a mild aniseed flavor to the dish.

1 Heat the oil over a moderately high heat. Stir-fry the fennel for about 3 minutes.

2 Add the salt and pepper to the flour and use this mixture to coat the livers.

3 Add the liver to the pan and cook it very quickly for about 5–10 minutes, stirring gently from time to time.

4 Slowly mix in the parsley and remove from heat. Pour in the vinegar. This should make a sizzling sound. Scrape the bits and juice from the pan and serve immediately.

MINI KABOBS WITH YOGURT DIP

These moist, beautifully flavored lamb kabobs make a great start to a meal. The yogurt dip is a traditional accompaniment, and is a cool, fresh contrast to the rich flavor of the meat. You could also serve this as a light lunch with pita bread and mixed salad.

1 Preheat the broiler to medium. Mix all the kabob ingredients together. As an alternative to lamb, you could use ground chicken or turkey.

2 With your fingertips, shape a level tablespoon (15 ml) of the meat mixture around each skewer, forming a sausage shape.

3 Broil the kabobs for 10–15 minutes until they are well browned, turning them frequently to make sure they cook through.

4 Meanwhile, make the dip by mixing all the ingredients together, and chill in the refrigerator until the kabobs are ready to serve.

FOR THE KABOBS

10½ oz (300 g) lean ground lamb

1 clove garlic, crushed

1 inch (2½ cm) ginger root, finely chopped

½ teaspoon (2 ml) salt

2 teaspoons (10 ml) paprika

FOR THE DIP

2 tablespoons (25 ml) chopped fresh mint

2 tablespoons (25 ml) chopped flat-leaf parsley

1 teaspoon (5 ml) cumin seeds

⅔ cup (150 ml) low-fat (1–2% M.F.) plain yogurt

Serves 4

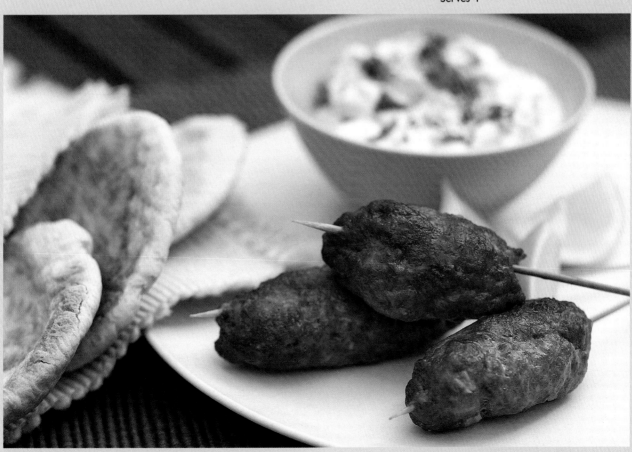

FALAFELS WITH MINT DIP

These crisp little savory balls originate from the Middle East, and make an unusual appetizer. These are baked rather than fried, so they are much lower in fat than the traditional version.

FOR THE FALAFELS

1 teaspoon (5 ml) coriander seeds

½ teaspoon (2 ml) cumin seeds

2 teaspoons (10 ml) olive oil

1 small onion, finely chopped

1 garlic clove, crushed

1¾ cups (425 ml) canned chickpeas, drained and rinsed

Large handful flat-leaf parsley, chopped

2 teaspoons (10 ml) all-purpose flour

Large pinch of salt

FOR THE DIP

1 teaspoon (5 ml) mint sauce

1 cup (250 ml) low-fat (1–2% M.F.) plain yogurt

Makes 12 falafels

1 Preheat the oven to 450°F (230°C). Put the coriander and cumin seeds in a small, dry frying pan and heat gently for 2–3 minutes until they become slightly brown and give off a fragrant smell.

2 Grind the seeds to a powder in a mortar and pestle or clean coffee grinder.

3 Heat the olive oil in the frying pan and fry the the onion and garlic for about 1–2 minutes, until they are softened.

4 In a bowl, mash the chickpeas to a pulp with a fork, leaving a few rougher pieces for texture. Add the ground roasted spices, onion and garlic mixture, chopped parsley, flour and salt.

5 Mix together well with your hands, and roll it into 12 small balls. Put these in an ovenproof dish and bake for 20 minutes.

6 Meanwhile, make the dipping sauce by mixing together the mint sauce and yogurt. Serve the falafels warm with the mint dip.

ROASTED BABY TOMATOES & EGGPLANT

Oozing with aromatic juices, these roasted vegetables are flavored with balsamic vinegar and make a colorful appetizer—they are best served with warm ciabatta bread.

4 baby eggplants, stalks trimmed

8 small plum tomatoes, pierced once

2 tablespoons (25 ml) balsamic vinegar

Salt and pepper, to taste

Serves 4

1 Preheat the oven to 375°F (190°C). Cut the baby eggplants into quarters lengthwise.

2 Put them into an open ovenproof dish with the tomatoes and drizzle them with the balsamic vinegar. Season, then roast in the oven for 1 hour.

ROASTED FENNEL & EGGPLANT

Cut 2 fennel bulbs into quarters and 2 small eggplants into bite-sized chunks. Lightly grease an ovenproof dish, season the vegetables well and bake in the oven at 375°F (190°C) for 30–40 minutes.

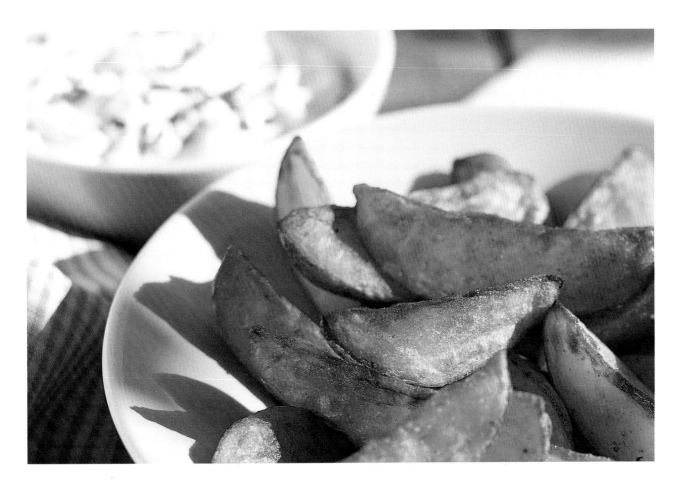

CRISPY POTATO WEDGES WITH CREAM & CHIVE DIP

These crunchy golden potato wedges are cleverly cooked so that they are healthily low in fat.

1　Preheat the broiler to high and line the broiler pan with aluminum foil.

2　Cut each potato lengthwise into 8 wedges. Boil in lightly salted water for 8–10 minutes or until they are just cooked. Drain.

3　Lightly grease the foil, and put the cooked potatoes onto the broiler pan. Season with the chili powder and salt and pepper to taste.

4　Drizzle or brush the oil over the potato wedges, place under a hot broiler and brown for 5–10 minutes.

5　Meanwhile, make the dip by mixing all the ingredients together. Serve the cooked wedges hot with the dip.

FOR THE POTATOES

3 baking potatoes (about 1 lb/454 g), scrubbed

2 tablespoons (25 ml) canola or olive oil

½ teaspoon (2 ml) chili powder

Salt and pepper, to taste

FOR THE DIP

2 tablespoons (25 ml) low-fat sour cream

6 oz (175 g) Balkan-style yogurt

⅓ cup (75 ml) snipped chives

Serves 4

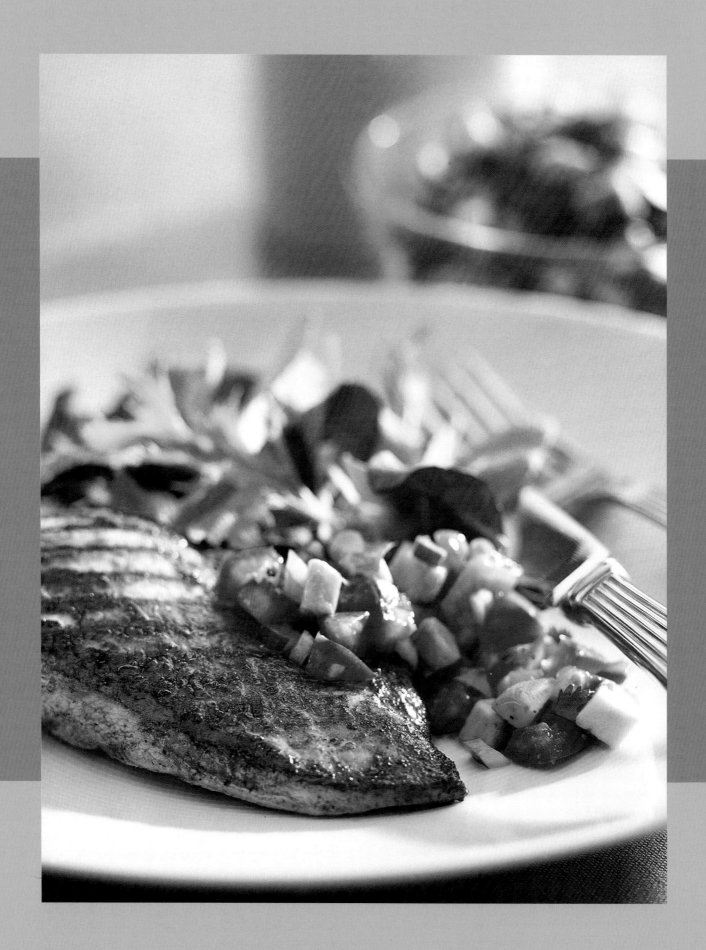

4 Main Meals

FISH
_____

POULTRY
_____

MEAT
_____

VEGETARIAN

TIGER SHRIMP RISOTTO

Non-fat cooking spray

---

1 small onion, peeled and finely chopped

---

4 small leeks, rinsed, trimmed and finely sliced

---

1 cup (250 ml) risotto rice, such as Arborio

3¾ cups (900 ml) hot stock made from equal parts of fish stock, chicken stock and water

---

14 oz (400 g) raw tiger shrimp, deveined and peeled

¾ cup (175 ml) frozen peas

¼ cup (50 ml) freshly grated Parmesan cheese

Serves 4

This fragrant risotto has a perfect texture—moist and creamy, with a satisfying "bite" to the rice. If you prefer, you can use cooked shrimp instead of raw—simply heat them through in the rice before serving.

1 Lightly spray a large, heavy-based saucepan. Add the onion and leeks and cook over medium heat until they are soft and translucent but not browned.

2 Add the rice and cook for 3 minutes stirring continuously, so that the grains are completely coated and slightly translucent.

3 Pour a ladleful of hot stock over the rice, stir and increase the heat so that the risotto bubbles gently. Stir continuously until the first batch of stock is absorbed. Continue adding and stirring in the stock, a ladleful at a time, until the rice is almost tender, but still *al dente,* or firm to the bite. Risotto should have a moist consistency, so, if necessary, add a little more stock.

4 Add the shrimp and peas and stir into the rice. Turn up the heat and cook for a further 5 minutes until the shrimp have cooked to a bright pink.

5 Remove from the heat, stir in the Parmesan cheese and serve immediately.

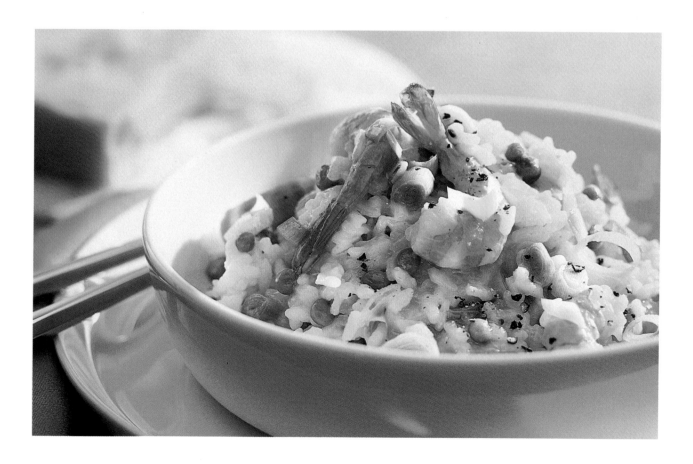

STIR-FRIED SQUID WITH LEMON GRASS & GINGER

Stir-fries are quick, healthy and hold the crisp textures of their fresh vegetable ingredients. Here, lemon grass and ginger add a sharp burst of flavor to succulent baby squid.

1   Preheat a wok, then add the sesame oil. Heat the oil until it starts to smoke.

2   Stir in the lemon grass and ginger, quickly followed by the red pepper and green onions.

3   Stir-fry for 1 minute, then add the squid, soy sauce and fish sauce, stirring continuously.

4   Cook for 4 minutes, toss in the bok choy and let it wilt slightly in the pan for a further minute. Add the egg noodles and mix well before serving.

1 tablespoon (15 ml) toasted sesame oil

2 stalks of lemon grass, outer leaves removed, finely chopped, then crushed with the blade of a knife

2 inch (5 cm) ginger root, peeled and finely chopped

2 small red bell peppers, seeded and diced

12 green onions, chopped

1 lb (454 g) baby squid, sliced into ½-inch (1 cm) rings

2 teaspoons (10 ml) soy sauce

½ teaspoon (2 ml) Thai fish sauce (nam pla)

4¼ cups (1050 ml) bok choy, ribs and leaves trimmed and roughly chopped

8 oz (225 g) medium egg noodles, cooked according to the package instructions

Serves 4

SMOKED FISH PARCELS

Smoked cod topped with a crunchy crust and baked in a foil parcel makes a fragrant treat—especially if you use naturally smoked fillets, which have a more subtle, delicate flavor than those dyed with artificial color. Serve with steamed new potatoes and baby carrots.

1   Preheat the oven to 375°F (190°C).

2   Cut a piece of aluminum foil 18" x 18" (45 cm x 45 cm), and spread it out flat. Place the green onions, button mushrooms and tarragon in the center, then add the pieces of smoked cod. Season with black pepper.

3   Mix the oatmeals together and press the mixture onto the flesh of the fish fillets to make a crust.

4   Turn the edges of the foil up, and pour the wine around the base of the fish. Seal the parcel with a double fold on the top and ends, leaving enough space for steam to expand.

5   Bake in the oven for half an hour, remove the tarragon and serve the fish on a bed of the baked onions and mushrooms.

6 green onions, chopped

6 oz (175 g) button mushrooms, sliced (about 2 cups/500ml)

Sprig of fresh tarragon

1 lb, 5 oz (600 g) smoked cod fillet, skinned and cut into 4 pieces

Black pepper, to taste

¼ cup (50 ml) quick-cooking oatmeal

2 tablespoons (25 ml) large flake rolled oats

¼ cup (50 ml) dry white wine

Serves 4

PAN-FRIED COD WITH PESTO

2 tablespoons (25 ml) olive oil

Salt and pepper, to taste

1¾ lb (800 g) cod fillets, skinned, and cut into 4 pieces

Juice of one fresh lime

FOR THE PESTO

4 tablespoons (60 ml) olive oil

2½ cups (625 ml) loosely packed fresh basil leaves

2 cloves garlic, peeled

½ cup (125 ml) pine nuts

3 tablespoons (45 ml) freshly grated Parmesan cheese

¼ cup (50 ml) cold water

Black pepper, to taste

Serves 4

Savor the aromatic scents, flavors and colors of Mediterranean cooking in this quickly prepared dish, and serve it with a fresh tomato salad and ciabatta bread. The pesto sauce is a low-fat version of the regional classic, and tastes just as good.

1 Heat a large, non-stick frying pan and add the olive oil. Season the cod fillets and pour half the lime juice over them. Pan-fry over medium heat, skin side down, and leave to cook for about 5 minutes.

2 Meanwhile, put the ingredients for the pesto into a blender and process until they are combined, but still retain a crumbly texture.

3 Turn the fillets and pour the remaining lime juice over them. Fry for another 4–5 minutes, until the fish is just cooked. Add a little cold water if the fish begins to stick to the pan.

4 Slide the cooked fillets gently onto a warmed serving dish, skin side down, and coat them with the pesto sauce. Serve immediately.

BALSAMIC SALMON STEAKS

4 salmon steaks, each about 6 oz (175 g)

FOR THE MARINADE

2 tablespoons (25 ml) balsamic vinegar

2 tablespoons (25 ml) soy sauce

1 tablespoon (15 ml) olive oil

2 teaspoons (10 ml) whole-grain mustard

2 garlic cloves, peeled and crushed

2 tablespoons (25 ml) fresh dill, finely chopped

Salt and pepper, to taste

Serves 4

Salmon is justly prized for its sweet flesh, and this imaginative recipe adds an intense, complex range of extra flavors. You can either soak the fish steaks in the rich, aromatic marinade, or cover them with the mixture and broil right away. Either way, they taste wonderful.

1 Place the salmon steaks in a non-metallic dish. In a separate bowl, mix together the vinegar, soy sauce, oil, mustard, garlic, dill and seasoning.

2 Pour the mixture over the salmon, turning it over to coat both sides. If marinating, cover the salmon and refrigerate for 30 minutes.

3 Preheat the broiler, and line the broiler pan with aluminum foil. Lift the salmon out of the marinade and place on the foil.

4 Broil under moderate heat for about 4–5 minutes each side, turning once.

GRILLED HALIBUT STEAKS WITH RED PEPPER SAUCE

If you're planning a special meal, try these tender steaks of halibut garnished with a spicy-sweet pepper sauce. Serve with wild rice, if available, and steamed green vegetables.

1 Preheat the broiler. Place the peppers skin side up on the broiler pan, and broil under high heat for about 15 minutes, or until the skins are blackened. Put them inside a plastic bag, and leave to cool for 10 minutes.

2 Meanwhile, line the broiler pan with aluminum foil. Brush the halibut steaks lightly on both sides with the olive oil, and spread the garlic and ginger over them. Season and put them on the broiler pan. Broil for 5–6 minutes on each side, turning once, until the flesh flakes easily. Remove

3 Make the sauce. Heat the oil in a frying pan and sauté the onions for about 2–3 minutes until they are translucent. Add the curry paste and cook for 1 minute.

4 Peel the peppers and put them in a food processor with the onion mixture, herbs, and lime juice. Blend until smooth and add seasoning if necessary.

5 Serve the fish with the red pepper sauce, garnished with lime wedges.

4 halibut steaks, about 6 oz (175 g) each

1 tablespoon (15 ml) olive oil

1 clove garlic, peeled and crushed

1 teaspoon (5 ml) chopped ginger root

Salt and pepper, to taste

FOR THE PEPPER SAUCE

2 teaspoons (10 ml) olive oil

1 small onion, chopped

1 teaspoon (5 ml) Thai red curry paste

3 red bell peppers, halved and seeded

Handful of fresh basil leaves, torn

Sprig of fresh thyme or a pinch of dried thyme

2 tablespoons (25 ml) lime juice

Lime wedges, to garnish

Serves 4

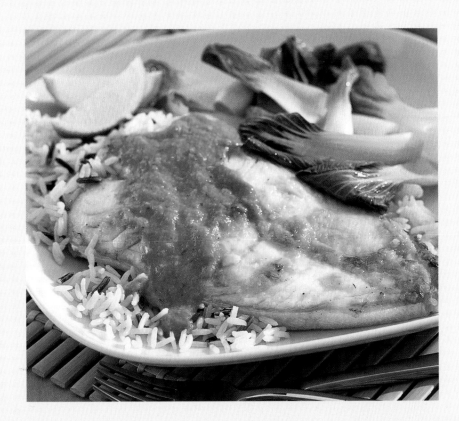

FETTUCCINE WITH SALMON, ASPARAGUS & LEMON

1 lb (454 g) fresh salmon fillets

12 oz (350 g) fresh fettuccine

10 fresh asparagus spears, cut in half

Juice of 2 large lemons

⅔ cup (150 ml) low-fat sour cream

¾ cup (150 ml) low-fat (1–2% M.F.) plain yogurt

Black pepper to taste

Fresh arugula leaves, to garnish

Serves 4

Pasta and salmon are perfect partners and this light, fragrant dish proves the point. Freshly cooked fettuccine is coated in a creamy, but healthily low-fat sauce studded with asparagus spears and salmon. All you need to serve it with is a simple salad of mixed leaves.

1   Preheat the oven to 375°F (190°C). Wrap the salmon in aluminum foil and bake for 30 minutes. Leave to cool for 10 minutes, remove any skin, and roughly flake the flesh. Set aside.

2   Meanwhile bring a large pan of lightly salted water to a boil, and cook the fettuccine for 2–3 minutes until *al dente*. Drain and set aside.

3   Simmer the asparagus spears gently for 5 minutes, then drain.

4   In a large saucepan, combine the lemon juice, sour cream and yogurt and cook over a low heat for 1–2 minutes.

5   Add the fettuccine, then fold in the asparagus spears and flaked salmon. Mix thoroughly and season with black pepper.

6   Serve immediately, garnished with fresh arugula leaves.

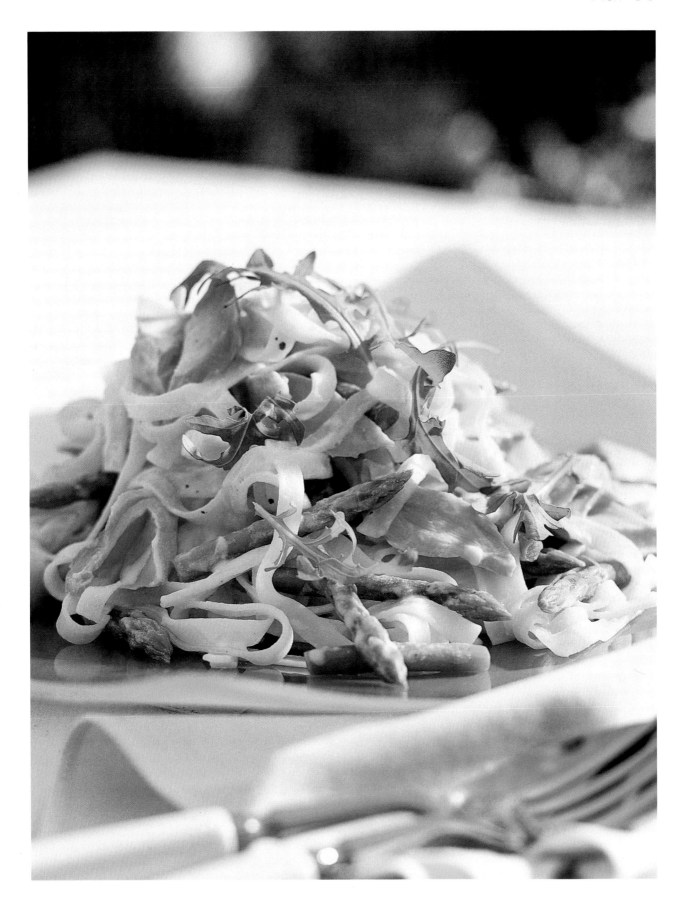

CORIANDER CHICKEN WITH ORANGE

Plump chicken thighs are scented with a medley of spices and citrus flavors. As the garlic cloves are cooked whole, they are not very pungent, and are soft and juicy to eat. The chicken is cooked on the bone, and makes a beautifully rich sauce that requires no extra thickening. Serve on a bed of rice or steamed couscous.

½ cup (125 ml) currants

⅞ cup (200 ml) unsweetened orange juice

1 tablespoon (15 ml) olive oil

4 large chicken thighs, skinned

1 large red onion, quartered and thickly sliced

4 whole garlic cloves, peeled

1 teaspoon (5 ml) coriander seeds, freshly crushed

2 medium red chili peppers, seeded and finely chopped

2 cinnamon sticks

⅓ cup (75 ml) whole blanched almonds

2 large oranges, peeled and white pith removed, roughly chopped

1¼ cups (300 ml) chicken stock

Sprigs of fresh mint, tied

Serves 4

1   Soak the currants overnight in half the orange juice, or for at least 1 hour.

2   Preheat the oven to 400°F (200°C). Heat the olive oil in a shallow, non-stick casserole dish and sauté the chicken for 2 minutes. Add the onions, garlic and coriander. Cook until the onions are soft and starting to brown.

3   Add the chili peppers, cinnamon sticks, almonds, currants, the remaining orange juice, chopped oranges, chicken stock and mint.

4   Bring to a boil, then transfer the casserole to the oven. Cook uncovered for 40 minutes. Discard the mint and cinnamon sticks and serve.

CHICKEN BREASTS WITH SALSA

The tangy salsa topping makes a splash of color on these tender chicken breasts and enhances the flavors of the peppery marinade. This is a relaxed, informal dish, ideal for eating outdoors. Serve it with rice and mixed vegetables, a mixed bean salad, tucked into pockets of warmed pita bread or folded inside tortilla wraps.

2 skinless, boneless chicken breasts each about 5 oz (150 g)

1 tablespoon (15 ml) corn or canola oil

FOR THE MARINADE

Juice of 1 lime

1 teaspoon (5 ml) tomato paste

1 tablespoon (15 ml) Worcestershire sauce

½ teaspoon (2 ml) cayenne pepper

1   Combine the marinade ingredients in an ovenproof dish and mix in the chicken breasts so they are completely coated. Refrigerate overnight, if possible, otherwise marinate for at least 1 hour.

2   Make the salsa. To loosen the skin from the tomatoes, make a small incision in the skin of each one, then plunge them into boiling water for 1 minute. Lift them out with a slotted spoon, and immediately plunge them into cold water. Leave them in the cold water for about 1 minute, then lift them out. Remove the skin from the tomatoes, chop the flesh finely and transfer to a bowl.

3 Add the remaining salsa ingredients and mix together thoroughly. Cover and leave aside to allow the flavors to develop.

4 Brush the surface of a non-stick grill pan or heavy-based frying pan with the oil and place over high heat until it is very hot. Add the chicken breasts and lower the heat to medium. Cook for 5–6 minutes on both sides until they are fully cooked and slightly charred. Serve hot with the salsa.

BARBECUED CHICKEN KABOBS

If you prefer, you can barbecue the chicken. Cut the breasts into cubes before marinating, then thread them onto skewers, adding alternating pieces of vegetables such as mushrooms, onions and peppers. Baste with the remaining marinade, and cook until the juices run clear when pierced with a knife.

FOR THE SALSA

2–3 large tomatoes

I large, ripe avocado, flesh removed and diced

I small red onion, finely diced

I cup (250 ml) fresh cilantro, chopped

Juice of I lime

Dash of hot pepper sauce, to taste

Salt and pepper, to taste

Serves 2

CHICKEN WITH GINGER

The luscious flavors of aromatic ginger combined with sweet honey and tangy lemons make this dish elegant enough for a dinner party. But it is also an inexpensive choice for a relaxed family occasion. Though honey is used here, it is less likely to make your blood glucose rise quickly when cooked with other ingredients.

1 Combine the ingredients for the marinade in a non-metallic dish that will hold the chicken comfortably. Using a sharp knife, make several deep cuts in the upper sides of the chicken breasts. Place them in the marinade, cut side down. Leave overnight, or for at least 4 hours, turning occasionally.

2 Preheat the oven to 375°F (190°C). Cut four pieces of aluminum foil 12" x 12" (30 cm x 30 cm), and brush with the sunflower oil.

3 Remove the chicken breasts from the marinade and wrap each one loosely in foil. Place the foil parcels on a non-stick baking tray.

4 Roast the chicken breasts in the center of the oven for 25 minutes or until they are cooked through (the juices should run clear when the chicken is pierced with a knife).

5 While the chicken is cooking, pour the remaining marinade into a small pan, add the cornstarch paste, and cook gently, stirring all the time, until the mixture thickens. Be sure the marinade is brought to a high heat and rapid boil. Season with salt and pepper to taste.

6 Unwrap the foil parcels and serve the chicken covered with the sauce, and garnished with the lemon zest.

FOR THE MARINADE

¾ cup (175 ml) freshly squeezed lemon juice

2½ tablespoons (37 ml) preserved ginger, finely chopped

I tablespoon (15 ml) liquid honey

2 cloves garlic, peeled and crushed

2 tablespoons (25 ml) dark soy sauce

FOR THE CHICKEN

4 skinless, boneless chicken breasts, each about 6 oz (175 g)

I tablespoon (15 ml) sunflower oil

2½ tablespoons (37 ml) cornstarch, mixed to a thin paste with a little water

Salt and pepper, to taste

2 teaspoons (10 ml) finely grated lemon zest, to garnish

Serves 4

CHICKEN WITH CARDAMOM

10 oz (300 g) skinless, boneless chicken breasts, chopped into bite-sized pieces

Cooking spray

8 whole black cardamom pods

1¼ inch (3 cm) stick cinnamon

1 bay leaf

4 whole cloves

2 small onions, finely chopped

¾ cup (175 ml) ground almonds

3 cloves garlic, peeled and crushed

1 inch (2½ cm) ginger root, peeled and coarsely grated

1 teaspoon (5 ml) ground cumin

1¼ cups (300 ml) low-fat (1–2% M.F.) plain yogurt

¾ cup (175 ml) chicken stock

⅔ cup (150 ml) raisins

1 tablespoon (15 ml) roasted whole almonds, ground or chopped very finely

Serves 4

Succulent pieces of chicken breasts are scented with a heady mix of fragrant spices. Serve with basmati rice cooked with a pinch of golden saffron, and a green vegetable such as steamed green beans. Black cardamom pods are widely available in Asian food stores, as well as supermarkets (green cardamom pods do not make a suitable substitute).

1 Choose a large, shallow, non-stick pan with a close-fitting lid, and spray the base with cooking spray. Heat gently, then add the chicken pieces.

2 Cook the chicken over low heat until it starts to color, stir in the whole spices and onions, and cook for 3–4 minutes.

3 Add the ground almonds, garlic, ginger and cumin and cook for a further 3 minutes. Pour in the yogurt and chicken stock gradually, stirring continuously while doing so.

4 Cover, reduce the heat to low, and cook gently for 20 minutes. Add the raisins, mix thoroughly, then cover and cook for another 10 minutes.

5 Remove the whole spices. Serve the chicken hot on a bed of rice, sprinkled with the crushed almonds.

TURKEY WITH RED ONION & WATERCRESS SALAD

FOR THE TURKEY

2 tablespoons (25 ml) all-purpose flour

1 teaspoon (5 ml) paprika

1 teaspoon (5 ml) Cajun seasoning

1 teaspoon (5 ml) Herbes de Provence

Salt and pepper, to taste

4 skinless, boneless turkey breasts, about 6 oz (175 g) each, cut into ½-inch (1-cm) wide strips

2 tablespoons (25 ml) corn or canola oil

Turkey breast has a more intense flavor than chicken, but is just as healthily low in fat. Skinless, boneless breasts are often available in convenient packages, and they are perfect for this tasty, char-grilled dish.

1 Mix the flour with the paprika, Cajun seasoning, herbs, and salt and pepper to taste. Use the mixture to coat the strips of turkey breast.

2 Pour the oil into a heavy-based non-stick frying pan, and place over high heat. Add the turkey strips, and lower the heat to medium.

3 Fry the turkey strips in the oil for 3–4 minutes, until they are crisp and golden.

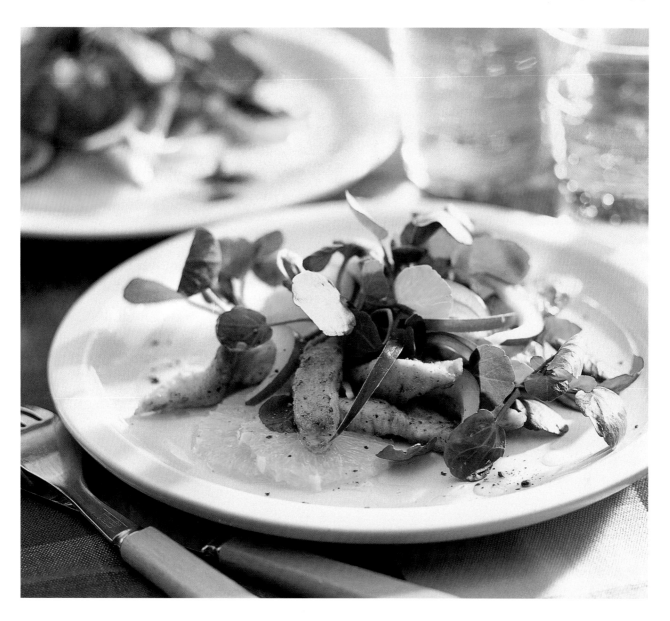

4   Meanwhile, make the salad. Mix together the watercress, red onion, lime juice and black pepper.

5   To serve, divide the turkey onto 4 warmed dinner plates. Arrange the orange slices on the side, and scatter the watercress salad on top.

FOR THE SALAD

1 large bunch fresh watercress, washed and trimmed

1 large red onion, sliced

Juice of 2 fresh limes

Black pepper, to taste

2 oranges, peeled, white pith removed and sliced into rounds

Serves 4

TURKEY FRICASSEE WITH OLIVE OIL MASHED POTATOES

FOR THE FRICASSEE

1 tablespoon (15 ml) all-purpose flour

Salt and pepper, to taste

2 tablespoons (25 ml) corn or canola oil

1 medium onion, finely chopped

2 cloves garlic, crushed

1 chicken bouillon cube

4 skinless, boneless turkey breasts (weighing about 6 oz (170 g) each), cut into bite-sized chunks

3 medium carrots, diced

1 green bell pepper, seeded and diced

½ cup (125 ml) Balkan-style yogurt

¼ cup (50 ml) fresh parsley, chopped

FOR THE MASH

1 lb (454 g) potatoes, peeled and chopped

½ teaspoon (2 ml) garlic salt, or to taste

⅔ cup (150 ml) skim milk

1 tablespoon (15 ml) low-fat cream cheese or sour cream

1 teaspoon (5 ml) Herbes de Provence

2 tablespoons (25 ml) extra virgin olive oil

Few sprigs fresh parsley

Serves 4

The traditional fricassee is a white stew of poultry and vegetables which are first fried in butter and then cooked in stock with the addition of cream and egg yolks. This recipe is adapted to keep the saturated fat down by using thick, Balkan-style yogurt and chicken stock to make an appetizing sauce for turkey, carrots and green peppers. It goes extremely well with soft Mediterranean mashed potatoes.

1   Mix the flour with the seasoning and use this to coat the turkey pieces.

2   Heat the oil in a non-stick pan. Add the onion and garlic and fry for a few minutes to soften them.

3   Make the chicken bouillon cube up to 1 cup (250 ml) with hot water.

4   Add the turkey to the pan and brown over a medium heat, adding a little of the stock if it sticks to the bottom.

5   Stir in the carrots and remaining stock. Cover and simmer for 5 minutes.

6   Meanwhile, boil the potatoes with the garlic salt until tender.

7   Add the green pepper to the fricassee and allow to cook, covered, for a further 5 minutes.

8   Stir in the yogurt and fresh parsley. Warm through over low heat and adjust the seasoning if necessary.

9   Drain and mash the potatoes with the milk, cheese or sour cream, herbs and olive oil. Serve hot with the fricassee and garnish with fresh parsley sprigs.

COD FRICASSEE
Use 4 medium fillets of cod instead of the turkey and cut them into bite-sized chunks. Coat them in the seasoned flour as above and fry with the onion and garlic until just cooked. Remove the fish and follow the method above until the fricassee is cooked through. Add the cooked fish to the yogurt and serve with the mash.

DUCK BREASTS WITH COCONUT

Flavored with spicy-sweet Thai curry paste and reduced-fat coconut milk (both available from large supermarkets and Asian food stores), these duck breasts are succulent and fragrant; serve them simply on a bed of steamed basmati rice. By removing the skin and surface fat, you reduce the fat content considerably.

1 Preheat the broiler to high, then place the duck slices on the broiler pan, and cook for about 4 minutes.

2 Warm the coconut milk in a wok or large, heavy-based frying pan, then add the curry paste and the snow peas. Simmer for one minute.

3 Stir in the duck, tomatoes and basil leaves, and simmer for 10 minutes more until the meat absorbs the flavors. Serve immediately.

10 oz (300 g) duck breasts, skin and surface fat removed, cut into ½-inch (1-cm) thick slices

1¼ cups (300 ml) reduced-fat coconut milk

2 teaspoons (10 ml) red Thai curry paste

1½ cups (375 ml) snow peas

12 cherry tomatoes, halved

Handful of fresh basil leaves

Serves 4

SWEET & SOUR DUCK

You can use fresh or canned pineapple in this easy version of a classic sweet and sour dish—both give excellent results. Serve with plain steamed rice or egg noodles.

1 Preheat the broiler to medium hot, and place the duck breasts on the broiler pan. Cook for about 5–6 minutes each side, depending on their thickness.

2 In a large saucepan, heat the sesame oil, then add the diced peppers and cook until they are softened.

3 Drain the juice from the pineapple and add the juice to the peppers. Mix in the wine vinegar, brown sugar, tomato paste, soy sauce, and sherry, then stir in the cornstarch paste. Continue stirring until the sauce is thick and glossy.

4 Add the grated carrot to the sauce, and cook for 3 minutes. Then add the pineapple pieces and cook for a further 2 minutes before serving. If the mixture becomes too thick, add a little more water.

5 Spoon the sweet and sour sauce onto a serving plate, and arrange the slices of duck breast over the top. Sprinkle with sesame seeds to garnish.

4 x 4 oz (115 g each) duck breasts, skin and surface fat removed

FOR THE SWEET AND SOUR SAUCE

1 teaspoon (5 ml) sesame oil

2 bell peppers (one red, one yellow), seeded and finely diced

1¾ cups (425 ml) fresh pineapple, diced and soaked in ⅔ cup (150 ml) unsweetened pineapple juice (or 14 oz/398 ml canned pineapple chunks)

¼ cup (50 ml) white wine vinegar

2 tablespoons (25 ml) light brown sugar

1 tablespoon (15 ml) tomato paste

3 tablespoons (45 ml) soy sauce

2 tablespoons (25 ml) dry sherry

2 tablespoons (25 ml) cornstarch, mixed to a thin paste with ½ cup (125 ml) water

1 large carrot, grated

1 tablespoon (15 ml) sesame seeds, to garnish

Serves 4

SMOKED SAUSAGE CASSOULET

Non-fat cooking spray

I garlic clove, peeled and crushed

12 small whole shallots, peeled

9 oz (250 g) fresh, lean spicy or garlic-flavored sausage, cut into chunks

3 oz (85 g) dried sausage such as Chorizo, cut into pieces

2 cups (500 ml) canned lima beans, drained

2¼ cups (550 ml) canned white kidney beans, drained

3 cups (750 ml) canned tomatoes

Pinch of mixed herbs

I tablespoon (15 ml) tomato paste

I tablespoon (15 ml) Dijon mustard

Salt and pepper to taste

2 tablespoons (25 ml) chopped parsley, to garnish

Serves 4–6

Traditionally a rustic French dish, this easy version makes a warming family meal on cold winter evenings. It's packed with flavor, and you'll need chunks of crusty French bread to soak up the juices. If you can't get shallots, use 3 small onions, peeled and cut into quarters. Accompany the cassoulet with lightly steamed cauliflower and broccoli florets.

1 Coat the base of a large saucepan with non-stick cooking spray. Cook the garlic and shallots (or onions if using) for 2–3 minutes over medium heat, until they are softened but not browned.

2 Add the fresh and dried sausage pieces and mix thoroughly. Cook for 5 minutes until the sausage is lightly colored, then add the beans, tomatoes, herbs, tomato paste, mustard and seasoning.

3 Bring the mixture to a boil, then reduce the heat. Cover and simmer gently for 20 minutes to allow the flavors to develop.

4 Sprinkle with the chopped parsley and serve immediately.

ITALIAN MEATBALLS

FOR THE MEATBALLS

14 oz (400 g) lean ground pork

¼ cup (50 ml) fresh bread crumbs

I egg white

I tablespoon (15 ml) pesto sauce

Salt and pepper, to taste

FOR THE TOMATO SAUCE

I small onion, finely chopped

I clove garlic, crushed

1¾ cups (425 ml) stewed canned tomatoes

¼ cup (50 ml) wine (red or white)

12 oz (350 g) penne, cooked *al dente*, to serve

Serves 4

Meatballs are a universal family favorite, originating from the south of Italy, and full of the sunny flavors typical of that region. These are made with healthily lean pork and are served with penne, but any pasta is suitable.

1 Preheat the oven to 375°F (190°C). In a large bowl, combine all the ingredients for the meatballs and mix them thoroughly with your hands.

2 Place the mixture on a square of waxed paper, and pat it out into a ¾-inch (2-cm) thick square. Cut it out into ¾-inch (2-cm) cubes, then, with wet hands, roll each cube into a firmly packed ball. This way, you'll get evenly sized meatballs.

3 Place the meatballs in a greased ovenproof dish and bake for 20 minutes.

4 Put the ingredients for the tomato sauce in a saucepan, and bring to a boil. Lower the heat, and simmer, uncovered, until the meatballs are ready.

5 Transfer the meatballs into the pan of tomato sauce and simmer for a further 10 minutes. Serve with the pasta.

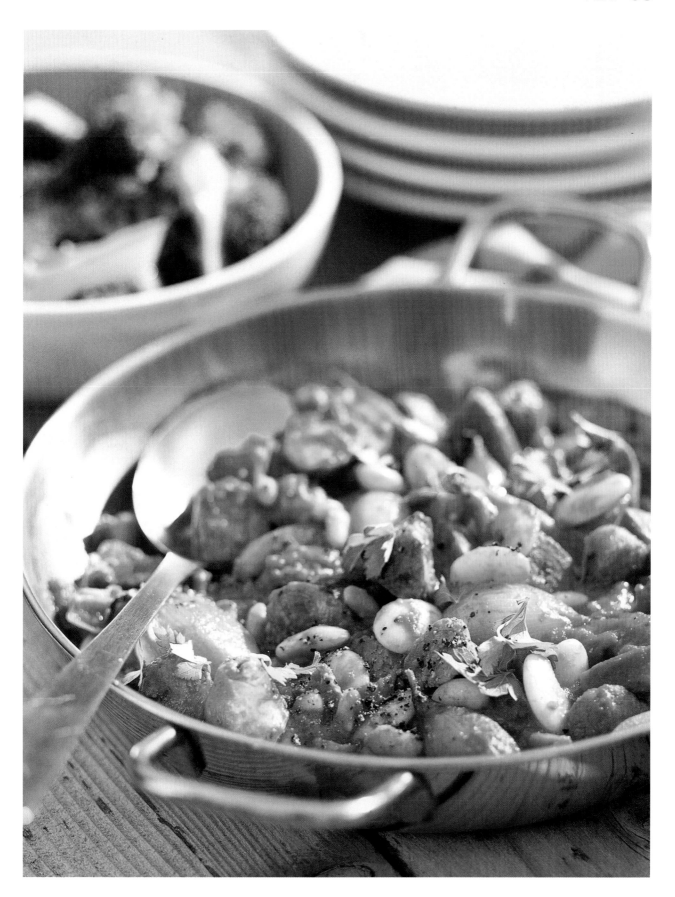

Beef with Green Pepper & Noodles

This tangy dish is delicious and cooks quickly once the meat is marinated, which can be done long beforehand. The beef is cut into thin strips so it takes very little time to cook. Noodles and other pasta have a low glycemic index and if you use rice noodles, you'll be going for an even lower fat option.

1 lb (454 g) flank steak, cut into thin strips across the grain

3 tablespoons (45 ml) soy sauce

1 tablespoon (15 ml) dry sherry

2 tablespoons (25 ml) vegetable oil

1 leek, trimmed, rinsed and thinly sliced into rings

1 green bell pepper, seeded, cut into chunks

1 inch (2½ cm) ginger root, peeled and sliced thinly

1 cup (250 ml) bean sprouts

2 large tomatoes, cut into wedges

2 teaspoons (10 ml) sesame oil

12 oz (350 g) fine egg or rice noodles (about 3 cups/750 ml dried)

Salt and pepper

Serves 4

1　Coat the meat well with the mixture of the soy sauce and the sherry. Leave to marinate for 30 minutes. Drain the beef, reserving the marinade.

2　Cook the noodles in a large saucepan of boiling water, following the instructions on the package. Drain and set aside.

3　Heat the oil in a wok and stir-fry the meat for 2–3 minutes on high. Remove with a slotted spoon and keep warm.

4　Add the leeks, pepper and ginger and stir-fry for 4 minutes. Next add the marinade, cooked beef and the bean sprouts. Cook for 2–3 minutes until the vegetables are cooked but crisp.

5　Heat the sesame oil in a wok or large pan. Stir in the noodles, season and serve with the beef.

Grilled Beef Tenderloin with Wild Mushrooms

A tantalizing mix of wild mushrooms and tender beef, all coated in a rich creamy sauce. Serve this with a pile of fresh vegetables such as broccoli or snow peas and balance it with some new boiled potatoes in their skins.

1 lb (454 g) beef tenderloin

2 tablespoons (25 ml) unsalted butter

1 medium onion, finely chopped

1 lb (454 g) wild mushrooms, sliced

1 tablespoon (15 ml) tomato paste

1 tablespoon (15 ml) Dijon mustard

2 tablespoons (25 ml) all-purpose flour, or as required

¼ cup (50 ml) low-fat sour cream

Salt and pepper

Serves 4

1　Wipe and trim the steak. Beat it flat and cut into bite-sized pieces.

2　Heat half the butter and fry the onions and mushrooms over a low heat until just beginning to color.

3　Stir in the tomato paste, mustard and enough flour to absorb the fat. Continue frying over a low heat for a couple of minutes, then carefully blend in the sour cream. Remove from heat.

4　Heat the remaining butter in a clean non-stick pan and fry the meat for a few minutes over high heat till brown. Add a little water if it sticks to the bottom.

5　Blend the beef into the sauce, season and serve.

LAMB WITH APRICOTS

Tender lamb and succulent apricots complement each other beautifully in this recipe, and produce a wonderfully rich, aromatic sauce. You'll need to soak this up with saffron-flavored rice, mashed potato or steamed couscous. Serve with some lightly steamed green beans or snow peas to give a fresh, green contrast.

1 Marinate the apricots, orange zest and raisins in the cider and orange juice for several hours or overnight.

2 Preheat the oven to 350°F (180°C). Spray the base of a large casserole pan with a thin layer of non-stick cooking spray, and brown the meat lightly.

3 Add the onion, mushrooms, pepper and garlic and cook for 5 minutes.

4 Add the stock, paprika, apricot mixture (including the marinade), bay leaves and Worcestershire sauce.

5 Cover and cook in the oven for 1 hour. Remember to remove the bay leaves before serving.

¾ cup (175 ml) dried apricots

Grated zest and juice of 1 orange

3 tablespoons (45 ml) seedless raisins

1⅔ cups (400 ml) dry cider

Non-stick cooking spray

14 oz (400 g) lamb tenderloin, trimmed and cut into ½-inch (1-cm) thick slices

1 large onion, chopped

1¼ cups (300 ml) button mushrooms

1 large yellow bell pepper, seeded and sliced

1 clove garlic, peeled and crushed

1¼ cups (300 ml) beef or lamb stock

Pinch of paprika

2 bay leaves

1 tablespoon (15 ml) Worcestershire sauce

Serves 4

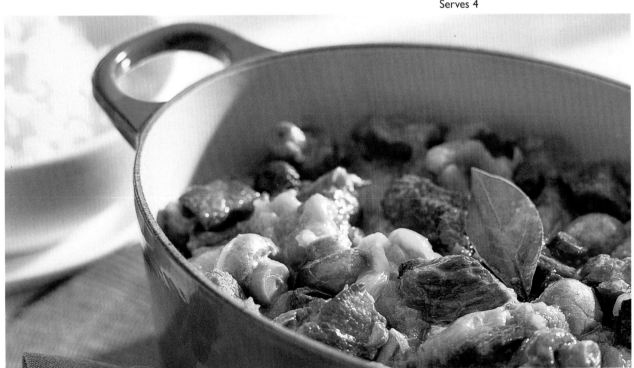

LAMB BAKED IN YOGURT

5 lbs (2¼ kg) leg of lamb, fat and skin removed

FOR THE MARINADE

¾ cup (175 ml) ground almonds

2 large onions peeled and coarsely chopped

8 cloves garlic, peeled

4 inch (10 cm) ginger root, peeled and chopped

4 green chili peppers, seeded and chopped

2 cups (500 ml) low-fat (1–2% M.F.) plain yogurt

2 tablespoons (25 ml) ground cumin

4 teaspoons (20 ml) ground coriander

½ teaspoon (2 ml) cayenne pepper

1 teaspoon (5 ml) salt

½ teaspoon (2 ml) garam masala

2 tablespoons (25 ml) low-fat (1–2% M.F.) plain yogurt sprinkled with a pinch ground cumin, to serve

Serves 6–8

Cook this delicious recipe for a special dinner party. Moist, succulent, leg of lamb is baked in a coating of creamy yogurt and aromatic spices. Vegetable Pilaf (see page 67) would be a perfect accompaniment.

1   Wipe the leg of lamb with a cloth and place it in a non-stick roasting pan. As you'll be marinating the lamb overnight you may wish to put it in another dish first, which will fit in your refrigerator.

2   Combine the ground almonds, onions, garlic, ginger and chili peppers with 3 tablespoons (50 ml) of the yogurt in a blender and purée to a smooth paste.

3   Put the remaining yogurt in a bowl, and stir in the paste mixture, ground cumin, coriander, cayenne pepper, salt and garam masala. Mix thoroughly.

4   With a small, sharp, knife, make deep slashes in the surface of the lamb, and push the yogurt mixture into the gashes. Spread the remaining mixture over the meat, ensuring it is all covered. Cover with plastic wrap and refrigerate for 24 hours.

5   Preheat the oven to 400°F (200°C). Remove the wrap and, if needed, transfer the lamb and sauce to a non-stick roasting pan. Cover the dish tightly with aluminum foil or a lid. Bake, covered, for 1½ hours, basting 2–3 times with the sauce. Uncover, and bake for a further 45 minutes. Remove from the oven and let the meat sit for 15 minutes in a warm place before serving with the yogurt and cumin.

VENISON IN RED WINE

1 tablespoon (15 ml) corn oil

1 lb, 5 oz (600 g) stewing venison, fat removed, diced into 1-inch (2.5-cm) cubes

1 large onion, chopped

3 medium tomatoes, skins removed (see page 56) and chopped

1 bouquet garni

Small piece of cinnamon stick

5 pickled walnuts, sliced

½ cup (125 ml) dry red wine

¾ cup (175 ml) strong beef stock

Serves 4

Venison is now widely available, and is an excellent alternative to beef. It is healthy, low in fat, and has a superb flavor. Serve this fragrant casserole with Parsnip Croquettes (see page 78), creamy mashed potatoes and a lightly cooked green vegetable. Pickled walnuts are available at gourmet specialty shops selling English products.

1   Preheat the oven to 350°F (180°C). Heat a large, non-stick flameproof casserole dish, add the oil and stir in the diced venison. Sauté for 2–3 minutes to lightly brown the meat.

2   Add the onions, tomatoes, bouquet garni, cinnamon, walnuts, wine and stock and mix together thoroughly.

3   Bake in the oven for 1½ hours, and serve immediately.

BROCCOLI & HERB PASTA

Use a single, fresh green vegetable for this pasta dish, as this keeps the flavor clean and distinctive. Broccoli is used here, but you could use any vegetable you like, such as zucchini, cauliflower, green beans or fava beans. Like the pasta, the vegetable should be cooked al dente.

1 Cook the pasta shells in a large pan of boiling salted water for about 12 minutes or until just tender, and drain them well.

2 While the pasta is cooking, steam the broccoli until it is cooked, but still has a firm "bite." Meanwhile, heat the oil in a large non-stick pan and sauté the onion and garlic over a gentle heat for about 5 minutes or until soft.

4 Add the tomatoes, herbs, broccoli and seasoning and mix gently but thoroughly. Mix in the cooked pasta and reheat if necessary and serve with a sprinkling of fresh basil and Parmesan cheese.

10 oz (300 g) dried pasta shells

2 cups (500 ml) broccoli florets

1 tablespoon (15 ml) canola oil

1 medium onion, finely chopped

2 cloves garlic, peeled and crushed

1½ cups (375 ml) canned chopped tomatoes

1 teaspoon (5 ml) oregano

Salt and pepper, to taste

2½ tablespoons (37 ml) freshly grated Parmesan cheese and a few chopped fresh basil leaves, to serve

Serves 4

VEGETABLE PILAF

Saffron gives this dish a beautiful yellow color, but if you prefer, you can use a pinch of turmeric instead. Peas are a suitable alternative to fava beans.

1 Drain the rice and set aside.

2 In a large saucepan, heat the oil gently, and sprinkle in the cumin seeds, stirring continuously for a few seconds.

3 Add the sliced onion, peppercorns, cloves, cinnamon and bay leaf, mix well then stir in the vegetables, salt and soaked rice.

4 Add the vegetable stock and saffron, bring to a boil, then reduce the heat.

5 Cover tightly and cook over a low heat for about 15–20 minutes, until all the water has been absorbed and the rice is done.

1¼ cup (300 ml) basmati rice, washed and soaked in water for 1 hour

1 teaspoon (5 ml) corn or sunflower oil

1 teaspoon (5 ml) cumin seeds

1 small onion, sliced

12 peppercorns, crushed

4 cloves

1 stick cinnamon

1 bay leaf

4 large carrots, finely diced

¾ cup (175 ml) frozen peas

1 cup (250 ml) frozen baby fava beans

2¾ cups (675 ml) broccoli florets

½ teaspoon (2 ml) salt

2½ cups (625 ml) vegetable stock (or water)

Few saffron threads

Serves 4

POLENTA WITH TOMATOES, PORCINI & GOAT CHEESE

½ cup (125 ml) sun-dried tomatoes (not packed in oil)

1 oz (30 g) porcini (dried mushrooms)

2 cups (500 ml) water

¾ cup (175 ml) instant polenta

1 tablespoon (15 ml) olive or canola oil

½ teaspoon salt

4 oz (125 g) goat cheese, crumbled

4 sprigs fresh basil, to garnish

Serves 2

Nothing could be more deceptively simple than this polenta recipe, but it is utterly sophisticated. Use the ready-cooked polenta, which is now widely available in large supermarkets. This makes a delicious lunch or supper dish.

1   Soak the sun-dried tomatoes and mushrooms for about 30 minutes in hot water to cover. Drain and reserve the soaking liquid.

2   Bring the water to a boil in a heavy-based saucepan. Add the salt and whisk in the polenta. Bring to a boil, stirring continuously, then reduce the heat and cook until thick and the polenta comes away from the sides of the pan, about 3–4 minutes.

3   Add the oil, tomatoes and mushrooms along with 1 tablespoon (15 ml) of the reserved liquid to the polenta. Stir together well and season to taste.

4   Finally, stir in the goat cheese and serve immediately, garnished with fresh basil.

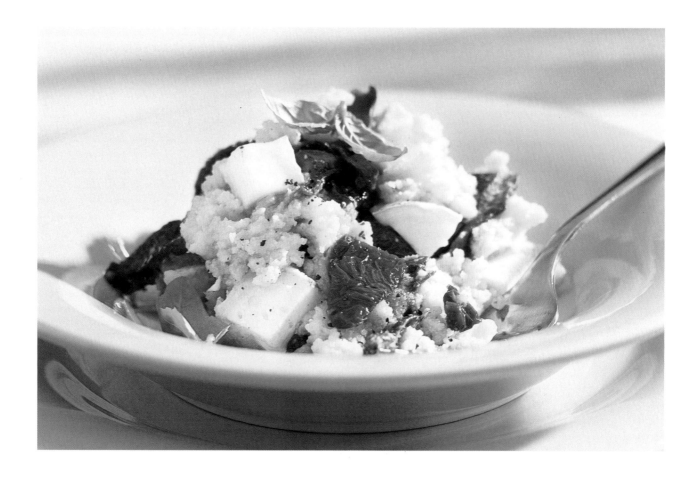

POLENTA BRUSCHETTA WITH MEDITERRANEAN VEGETABLES

Made from cornmeal, polenta has a distinctive golden color and is a popular dish from Northern Italy. As the traditional method requires long cooking, use instant polenta—it's widely available in supermarkets. These delicious bruschettas are flavored with Parmesan cheese, and topped with sunny Mediterranean vegetables.

1 Cook the polenta according to the package instructions. Once it comes to a boil, stir vigorously with a wooden spoon for about 5 minutes.

2 Add the Parmesan cheese, season to taste, and turn into a shallow, lightly oiled dish and allow to set.

3 Meanwhile, cook the vegetables. Heat the oil in a medium-sized pan, add the onion and sauté gently for 2–3 minutes until softened but not browned.

4 Add the green pepper, zucchini and eggplant and sauté for a further 5 minutes. Add the tomatoes, herbs and seasoning. Bring to a boil, then lower the heat and simmer, uncovered, until the vegetables are tender, but not mushy.

5 To make the bruschetta, preheat the broiler or grill. Cut the set polenta into 4 wedges or 12 slices and brush them with a little olive oil. Broil or grill until golden.

6 Serve covered with the vegetables, garnished with fresh basil leaves.

FOR THE BRUSCHETTA

8 oz (225 g) instant polenta

2½ tablespoons (37 ml) freshly grated Parmesan cheese

Salt and pepper, to taste

1 tablespoon (15 ml) extra virgin olive oil

Sprigs of fresh basil, to garnish

FOR THE TOPPING

1 tablespoon (15 ml) extra virgin olive oil

1 large onion, peeled and chopped

1 green bell pepper, seeded and roughly chopped

8 small zucchini, trimmed and sliced about ½-inch (1-cm) thick

3 baby eggplants, roughly chopped

1½ cups (375 ml) canned chopped tomatoes with garlic

1 teaspoon (5 ml) Herbes de Provence

Salt and pepper, to taste

Serves 4

MIXED-PEPPER COUSCOUS

Couscous, made from semolina, is a good alternative to potatoes, rice or pasta. This version is infused with the aromatic juices of peppers, onions and cilantro, and is delicious served with a little balsamic vinegar drizzled over it.

1 Put the dry couscous in a large mixing bowl, add the boiling water and mix briefly with a fork.

2 Stir in the olive oil and lime juice, add the chopped peppers, onion and cilantro, and mix together thoroughly.

3 Leave for 30 minutes for the flavors to develop, then serve.

8 oz (225 g) couscous

1¼ cups (300 ml) boiling water

2 tablespoons (25 ml) olive oil

Juice of 1 lime

3 small bell peppers (green, yellow and red), seeded and finely chopped

1 small red onion, finely chopped

2 cups (500 ml) fresh cilantro, roughly chopped

Serves 4

SPICY CHICKPEAS IN WHOLEWHEAT WRAPS

Homemade flat bread has a wonderful flavor, and it's not at all difficult to make. It's really versatile too—you can use it as a wrap for this tasty chickpea (garbanzo) filling, or as a flat bread, to use with dips and other accompaniments.

FOR THE WRAPS

4 cups (1 liter) wholewheat flour

Pinch of salt

1 cup (250 ml) lukewarm water

¼ cup (50 ml) vegetable oil

FOR THE FILLING

Cooking spray

1 small onion, finely chopped

Small piece of ginger root, peeled and grated

¾ cup (175 ml) canned tomatoes, chopped

1 green chili pepper, seeded and finely chopped

½ teaspoon (2 ml) turmeric

2 teaspoons (10 ml) ground coriander

½ teaspoon (2 ml) garam masala

½ teaspoon (2 ml) chili powder

1½ cups (375 ml) chickpeas, drained and rinsed

FOR THE SAUCE

1 tablespoon (15 ml) chopped cilantro

¼ cup (50 ml) low-fat (1–2% M.F.) plain yogurt

Serves 4 (makes 8 wraps)

1   Sift the flour and salt together. Gradually add the warm water and vegetable oil through your fingers and knead thoroughly into a stiff and pliable dough. Leave aside for half an hour to rest.

2   Heat a large saucepan and coat the base with cooking spray. Add the onion and ginger, and sauté until brown. Stir in the tomatoes, green chili pepper, turmeric, ground coriander, garam masala and chili powder and mix well.

3   Add in the chickpeas and add a little water if necessary. Reduce the heat and simmer gently for 10 minutes.

4   Meanwhile, break off a piece of the dough (about the size of a walnut) and shape into a smooth ball. Flatten the ball slightly, then roll out into a thin circle, about 8 inches (20 cm) in diameter.

5   Heat a heavy-based frying pan and place the dough on the hot surface. Cook one side until brown, then turn over to cook on the other side. Finally, turn the bread again, and lightly press around the edges with a clean cloth, so that it puffs up.

6   Keep the finished breads warm by wrapping them in aluminum foil or a cloth and put them to one side while you make the rest.

7   To make the serving sauce, mix the cilantro into the yogurt and stir thoroughly.

8   Divide the chickpea mixture into eight. Spoon one portion down the middle of each bread and carefully fold over the sides of the bread, securing with a toothpick, if necessary. Serve wraps with the yogurt sauce on the side or as a dip.

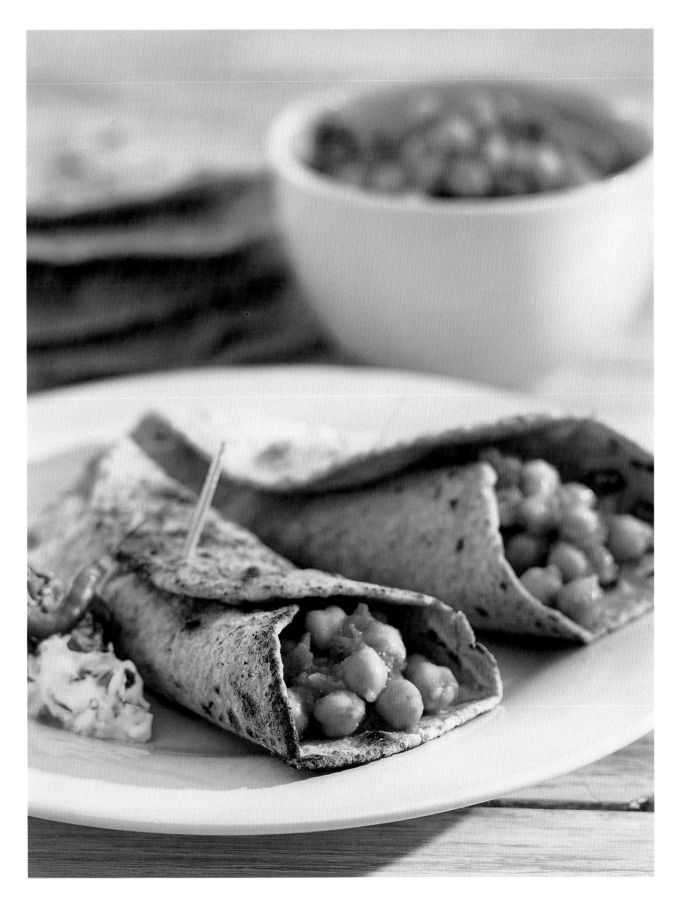

CREPES STUFFED WITH SPINACH & RICOTTA

FOR THE CREPES

2 cups (500 ml) chickpea flour

1 cup (250 ml) skim milk

1 cup (250 ml) water

Pinch of salt

Cooking spray

FOR THE FILLING

4½ cups (1125 ml) baby spinach leaves, rinsed

¾ cup (175 ml) ricotta cheese

¼ teaspoon (1 ml) nutmeg, freshly grated

2½ tablespoons (37 ml) Parmesan cheese, grated, to serve

Handful of fresh basil leaves, to garnish

Serves 2–4

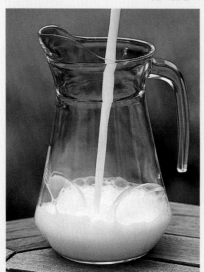

Once you've learned to make crepes successfully, you can experiment with various fillings. The spinach and ricotta combination suggested here, however, is a true classic. Serve with a hearty mixed salad. Chickpea flour is available at specialty food shops, particularly East Indian, Middle Eastern and some bulk-food stores. Use a 10–11 inch (25 cm) nonstick crepe pan.

1   To make the batter, put the chickpea flour and salt in a bowl, pour in the water and milk, and mix together thoroughly. Set aside.

2   Make the filling. Put the damp rinsed spinach in a saucepan without adding any extra water, and cook over medium heat for a minute or two until wilted. Turn off heat. Leave to cool slightly, drain well and chop. Add the ricotta and nutmeg and mix well. Set aside.

3   Choose a large, heavy-based frying pan, and coat with a few sprays of cooking spray. Place over high heat until it is hot.

4   Remove the pan from the heat. Pour in 2–3 tablespoons (25–45 ml) of batter, tipping the frying pan as you pour it in, so that the batter covers the base.

5   Return the pan to the heat and cook for about 30 seconds until the batter has started to set on top and is golden underneath. Loosen the edges of the crepe with a thin spatula, then flip it over, and cook the other side until golden. Keep the finished crepes warm by wrapping them in aluminum foil while you make the rest.

6   Before filling the crepes, warm the spinach and ricotta mixture over low heat, or heat in the microwave for 2 minutes. Evenly distribute the filling among the crepes, then fold one side over the other. Serve with a little grated Parmesan cheese and garnish with the basil leaves.

PENNE WITH ROASTED VEGETABLES

Roasted Mediterranean vegetables, fragrant with the aroma of fresh garlic, add brilliant color and flavor to the pasta. This delicious Italian meal will become a family favorite—serve it with a simple green salad and some crusty ciabatta bread.

1 Preheat the oven to 475°F (240°C). Drizzle a teaspoon (5 ml) of oil into a large roasting pan, then layer the red and yellow peppers and zucchini into the pan, adding the herbs and seasoning in between the layers. Drizzle most of the remaining oil over the vegetables, reserving about 2 teaspoons (10 ml).

2 Bake uncovered at the top of the oven for 20–25 minutes, until slightly charred, adding the tomatoes after 15 minutes. Stir once during cooking.

3 Cook the pasta in lightly salted water according to the package instructions until *al dente* (about 10 minutes).

4 Meanwhile, heat the remaining oil in a large non-stick frying pan. Add the garlic, onion and green pepper and fry until the onions are light brown and the peppers are just cooked.

5 Take the vegetables out of the oven, stir gently and mix thoroughly with the pasta, adjust the seasoning if necessary, and sprinkle with parsley.

3 tablespoons (45 ml) olive oil
I red bell pepper, seeded and diced
I yellow bell pepper, seeded and diced
3 medium zucchini, sliced thinly and diagonally
1½ teaspoons (7 ml) dried oregano
2 bay leaves
Salt and pepper to taste
3 medium, ripe tomatoes, cut into eighths
2½ cups (625 ml) penne
3 cloves garlic, peeled and crushed
I small onion, finely chopped
I green bell pepper, diced
I tablespoon (15 ml) finely chopped fresh parsley

Serves 4

SAFFRON RICE WITH VEGETABLES & SOFT HERB CREAM CHEESE

A colorful dish made from rice and vegetables—a perfect vegetarian meal with no need for any accompaniments. When combined, cream cheese and rice provide the protein in this balanced dish.

1 Heat the oil in a large saucepan with a lid. Fry the onions for about 5 minutes, until they are browned.

2 Add the stock, rice, vegetables, saffron and turmeric. Bring to a boil, lower the heat, cover and cook for 20 minutes, until the water is absorbed and the rice is done.

3 Preheat the grill to medium. Lightly grease a flameproof dish and place the cooked rice into this dish.

4 Cover the rice with a topping of low-fat cream cheese with herbs. Grill for about a minute and serve immediately.

I tablespoon (15 ml) corn oil
I medium onion, finely chopped
2 vegetable stock cubes, made up to 2 cups (500 ml) with boiling water
1¼ cups (300 ml) long grain rice
I lb (454 g) frozen mixed vegetables (about 4 cups/I liter)
Few strands of saffron
½ tsp (2 ml) ground turmeric
4 oz (115 g) low-fat cream cheese with herbs (about ⅓ cup/75 ml)

Serves 4

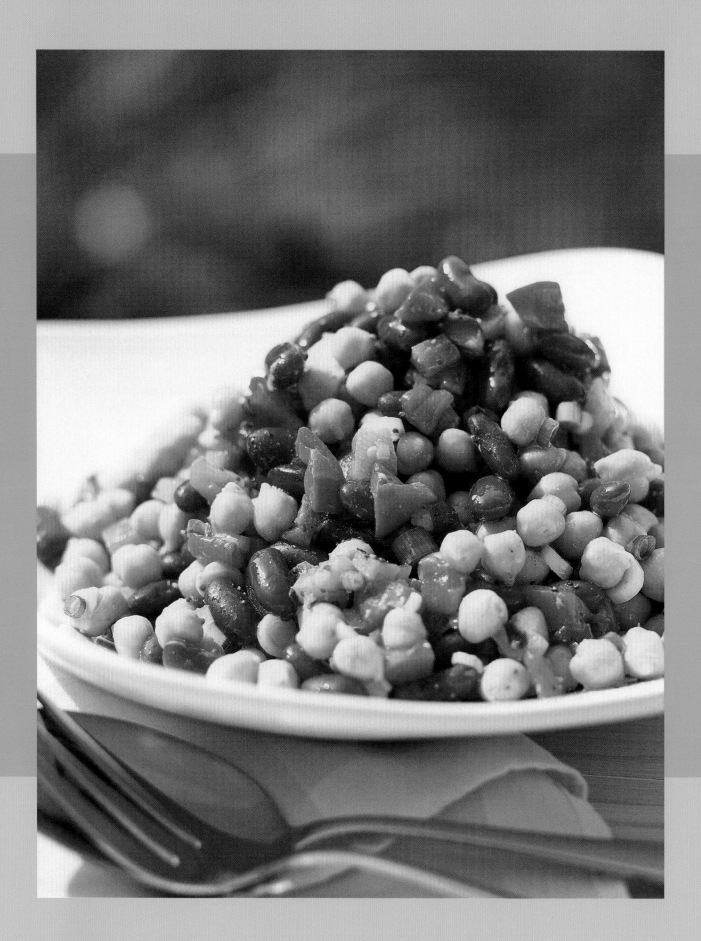

5

Vegetables & Side Dishes

POTATOES & ROOT VEGETABLES

CORN

MEDITERRANEAN VEGETABLES

LEGUMES & GREENS

LEMON & ONION ROASTED POTATOES

4–5 large baking potatoes (about 2 lbs/1 kg)

2 tablespoons (25 ml) olive oil

2 medium red onions, peeled and cut into quarters

1 large lemon (or 2 small lemons), cut into 6 wedges

Salt and pepper, to taste

Serves 4

These roast potatoes are bursting with aromatic flavors and make a perfect accompaniment to grilled meat and fish.

1   Preheat the oven to 325°F (160°C).

2   Peel the potatoes. Cut into equal-size pieces for roasting, and dry them thoroughly on paper towels.

3   Arrange the potatoes on a roasting pan and drizzle with the olive oil.

4   Add the wedges of onions and lemons and mix the vegetables together, keeping the onion pieces as whole as possible.

5   Season well. Roast for 1–1½ hours until the potatoes are crisp and golden.

ROASTED NEW POTATOES WITH TOMATOES & HERBS

1 lb (454 g) small new potatoes in their skins, washed and dried

1 tablespoon (15 ml) olive oil

2 bay leaves

2 large tomatoes, cut thickly into slices

Salt and pepper, to taste

1 teaspoon (5 ml) fresh thyme, finely chopped (or large pinch dried)

1 teaspoon (5 ml) fresh oregano, finely chopped (or large pinch dried)

Serves 4

Baby new potatoes are just the right size for roasting in their skins, and these are deliciously scented with tomatoes and fresh herbs. They are particularly good as an accompaniment to roast lamb.

1   Preheat the oven to 375°F (190°C). Cover the potatoes with boiling water and partially boil them for 3–5 minutes.

2   Make small cuts on each potato and arrange on a large roasting pan.

3   Add the olive oil, bay leaves, tomatoes, seasoning and herbs.

4   Toss roughly so that the potatoes and tomatoes are well coated, and bake in the oven for 40 minutes. Shake the pan occasionally during cooking.

ROASTED NEW POTATOES WITH HONEY & MUSTARD
After step 1, toss the potatoes in 2 tablespoons (25 ml) whole-grain mustard mixed with 2 tablespoons (25 ml) liquid honey, and 1 tablespoon (15 ml) olive oil. Season to taste, and bake in the oven for 40 minutes.

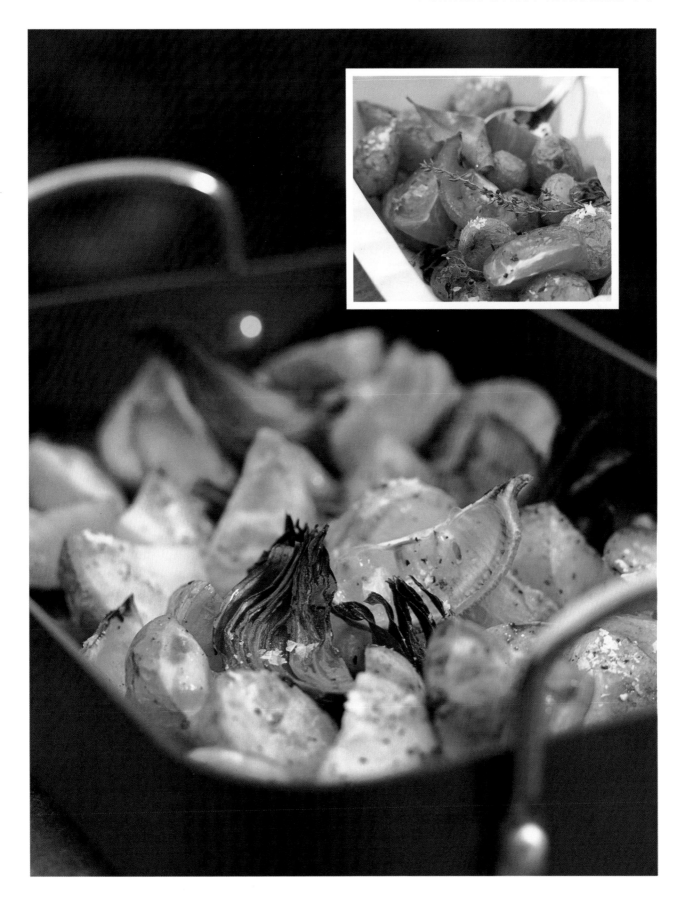

Baked Sweet Potatoes with Spicy Butter

4 large sweet potatoes

1 tablespoon (15 ml) butter
(or low-fat margarine)

Large pinch chili powder

Serves 4

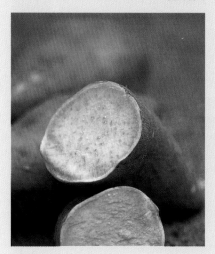

The potatoes ooze a sticky, delicious-tasting juice as they cook, so always roast them on a baking tray rather than a rack.

1 Preheat the oven to 400°F (200°C). Wash and dry the sweet potatoes and make 2–3 deep slashes into each of them.

2 Line a baking tray with parchment paper or aluminum foil and arrange the sweet potatoes on it. Bake them in the oven for 40–50 minutes until they are soft.

3 Meanwhile, make the spicy butter. In a bowl, mix together the butter (or low-fat margarine if using) and the chili powder.

4 Place the mixture onto a piece of plastic wrap, roll it into a small sausage shape and then chill in the refrigerator until the potatoes are cooked.

5 When the potatoes are soft, slit them open along the top surface and spoon a quarter of the spicy butter into each one. Serve immediately.

Parsnip Croquettes

FOR THE PARSNIPS

2 cups (500 ml) mashed potatoes

1½ cups (375 ml) cooked parsnips, mashed

¼ teaspoon (1 ml) ground cinnamon

¼ teaspoon (1 ml) ground nutmeg

FOR THE COATING

1 egg, beaten

Bread crumbs, as required

Makes 20 croquettes

These tasty morsels have a sweeter flavor than potato croquettes, and are special enough to serve as a side dish when you're entertaining. Use a little skim milk to mash the potatoes.

1 Preheat the oven to 375°F (190°C).

2 In a large bowl, mix together the potato mixture, parsnips and ground spices. Using your hands, shape the mixture into small croquettes about 1½ inches (3½ cm) long. Place the croquettes in the freezer for 5 minutes to chill.

3 Roll each croquette in the beaten egg, then in the bread crumbs, and place in an ovenproof dish. Bake, uncovered, for 30 minutes.

CORN FRITTERS

These golden fritters are very easy to cook, and make a tasty vegetable
accompaniment to a family meal. You can vary the flavor by adding
a handful of finely chopped fresh herbs or half a teaspoon (2 ml) of
finely chopped fresh chilies.

1 Preheat the oven to 375°F (190°C). Make the batter first, by sifting the flour
and salt together into a large bowl. Break the egg into the middle of the
flour and add the milk. Mix well, but do not beat. Leave the batter to rest
in the refrigerator for 30 minutes.

2 Add the corn to the batter, and mix thoroughly.

3 Heat a heavy-based, lightly greased non-stick frying pan until it is hot and
drop 1 tablespoon (15 ml) of the mixture for each fritter onto the hot surface. It is best to cook the fritters in batches of 3 or 4.

4 Bubbles will appear on the uncooked surface of each fritter. When these
burst, turn the fritter over and cook the other side until it is golden brown.
Brush the fritters with a little oil if they are sticking to the surface.

5 Drain them on paper towels to absorb any excess oil, and keep the cooked
fritters warm in the oven until all of them are ready. Serve hot.

1 cup (250 ml) all-purpose flour

⅓ cup (75 ml) skim milk

¼ teaspoon (1 ml) salt

1 large egg

1¾ cups (425 ml) canned corn, drained

Makes 15 fritters

STIR-FRIED BABY CORN & SNOW PEAS

Sesame oil and hulled sunflower seeds add a distinctive rich, nutty
flavor and crunchy texture to this crispy-fresh stir-fry.

1 Heat a wok to high temperature, then add the sesame oil. When the oil is
smoking, add the corn pieces, snow peas and green onions, and stir-fry for
3 minutes.

2 Sprinkle with the sunflower seeds, mix thoroughly and serve.

1 teaspoon (5 ml) sesame oil

1¾ cups (425 ml) canned baby corn cobs, halved

1⅓ cups (325 ml) snow peas

8 green onions, trimmed and chopped into 1-inch (2-cm) pieces

⅓ cup (75 ml) roasted unsalted sunflower seeds

Serves 4

SESAME-FRIED GREEN BEANS
Quickly steam 1 lb (454 g) green beans until they are still firm but just cooked.
Stir-fry 2 tablespoons (25 ml) of sesame seeds in 1 teaspoon (5 ml) of sesame oil
for ½ minute, add the drained beans, cook for a few more seconds and serve
immediately.

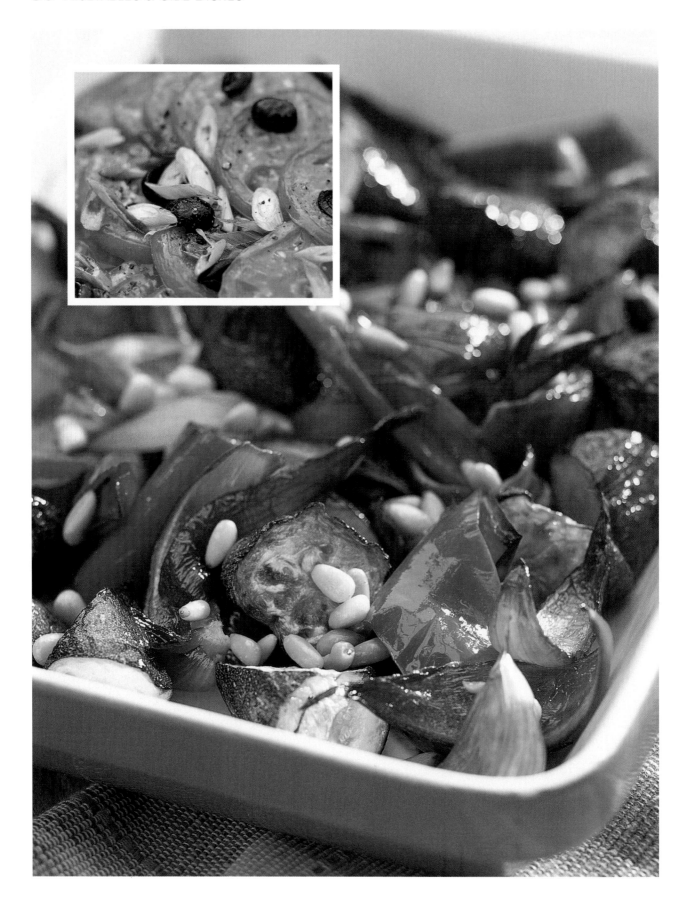

ROASTED MEDITERRANEAN VEGETABLES WITH PINE NUTS

A simple yet effective side dish that works very well served over rice or couscous.

1 Preheat the oven to 375°F (190°C). Drizzle the olive oil into a large, ovenproof casserole dish and warm it in the oven for about 5 minutes until it is hot.

2 Add the peppers, garlic, zucchini and onion, and mix well until all the vegetables have a light coating of oil. Roast in the oven for 30–40 minutes.

3 Meanwhile, toast the pine nuts. Heat a frying pan over medium heat and add the pine nuts. Shake the pan occasionally to move the nuts around, and toast them for 2–3 minutes until they are golden brown all over.

4 Serve the vegetables with the pine nuts sprinkled over them.

2 tsp (10 ml) olive oil

3 medium sweet, red bell peppers, seeded and roughly chopped

4 whole garlic cloves, unpeeled

8 small zucchini, sliced

1 large red onion, peeled and roughly chopped

⅓ cup (75 ml) pine nuts

Serves 2

BAKED TOMATO & OLIVE SALAD

Tomatoes are a delicious, versatile ingredient and a good source of antioxidants. Here, they are mixed with olives, making this an ideal accompaniment to grilled fish.

1 Preheat the oven to 400°F (200°C). Lightly grease an ovenproof dish.

2 Layer the tomatoes and the olives in the dish, and season with the paprika and garlic salt.

3 Drizzle the olive oil over the tomatoes and olives, and bake in the middle of the oven for about 15 minutes, until the tomatoes are soft but not mushy.

4 Garnish with the green onions and serve warm.

8 large tomatoes, sliced

12 black olives, halved and pitted

Paprika and garlic salt, to taste

1 tablespoon (15 ml) olive oil

2 green onions, trimmed and finely sliced

Serves 4

Tabouleh

FOR THE SALAD

¾ cup (175 ml) bulgur, presoaked in hot water for 1 hour, then drained

1¾ cups (425 ml) flat-leaf parsley, roughly chopped

5 medium tomatoes, diced

½ cup (125 ml) fresh mint leaves, finely chopped, or 2 tablespoons (25 ml) dried mint

1 medium onion, finely chopped

FOR THE DRESSING

Pinch of salt

Pinch of ground allspice

Pinch of ground cinnamon

Juice of 2 lemons

2 tablespoons (25 ml) olive oil

Serves 4

This is a delightfully light, fresh-tasting salad from the Middle East. You could serve it with grilled lamb kabobs, or as an accompaniment to grilled fish.

1   In a bowl, mix together the bulgur, parsley, tomatoes, mint and onion.

2   Make the dressing. Put all the dressing ingredients into a screw-top jar and shake vigorously.

3   Toss the bulgur mixture in the dressing, and serve.

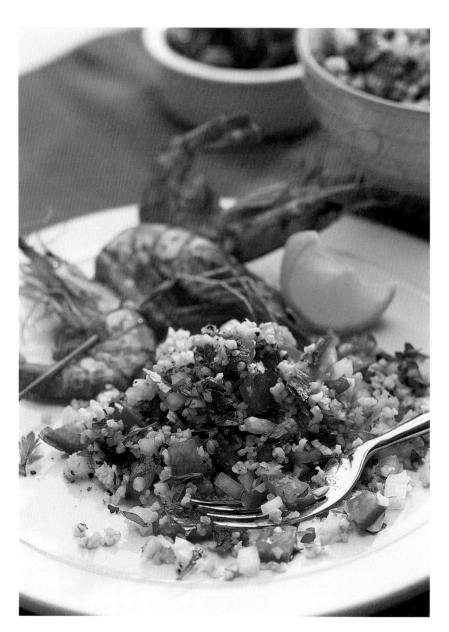

PEPPERY BEAN SALAD

This colorful salad is packed with flavor, and goes well with grilled fish; alternatively, it could make a delicious vegetarian dish—serve it with warmed pita bread to mop up the fragrant dressing.

1 Preheat the broiler. Place the peppers skin side up on the broiler tray, and cook under high heat for about 15 minutes, or until the skins are blackened. Put them inside a plastic bag, and leave to cool for 10 minutes.

2 Peel the peppers, then dice the flesh and place in a large bowl. Add the green onions, kidney beans and chickpeas, and mix.

3 Put all the dressing ingredients into a screw-top jar, and shake vigorously. Pour the dressing over the salad, and mix well.

4 Cover with plastic wrap and chill for at least 15 minutes before serving.

FOR THE SALAD

I red bell pepper, halved and seeded

I green bell pepper, halved and seeded

4 green onions, trimmed and finely chopped

1⅛ cups (275 ml) canned red kidney beans, drained and rinsed

1¾ cups (425 ml) canned chickpeas, drained and rinsed

FOR THE DRESSING

1½ tablespoons (22 ml) olive oil

Juice of I small lemon

I clove garlic, peeled and crushed

2 teaspoons (10 ml) whole-grain Dijon mustard

Serves 4

CABBAGE WITH CARAWAY SEEDS

Lightly steamed, and scattered with delicately flavored caraway seeds, this is the perfect way to prepare cabbage. Serve it with grilled lamb chops or thin slices of roast beef.

1 Steam the cabbage for 2–3 minutes until it is just cooked, but still a little firm. Drain thoroughly.

2 Heat the oil in a wok until it is smoking, add the cabbage, caraway seeds and seasoning and stir-fry for 2–3 minutes. Sprinkle on some cayenne pepper and serve immediately.

I lb (454 g) green cabbage, sliced

I tablespoon (15 ml) olive oil

2 tablespoons (25 ml) caraway seeds

Salt and pepper, to taste

Pinch of cayenne pepper

Serves 4

RED CABBAGE COLESLAW

The reduced-calorie mayonnaise in this side dish helps to keep the fat lower than in a standard coleslaw. If you want it even lower in fat, choose a low-fat natural yogurt or fat-free vinaigrette instead.

Simply mix all the ingredients together in a bowl and serve. If you are not eating this immediately, cover the bowl and keep it in the refrigerator until it is ready to serve.

½ lb (225 g) red cabbage, shredded or grated

3 medium carrots, grated

3 green onions, trimmed and sliced

½ cup (125 ml) low-fat mayonnaise

Serves 4

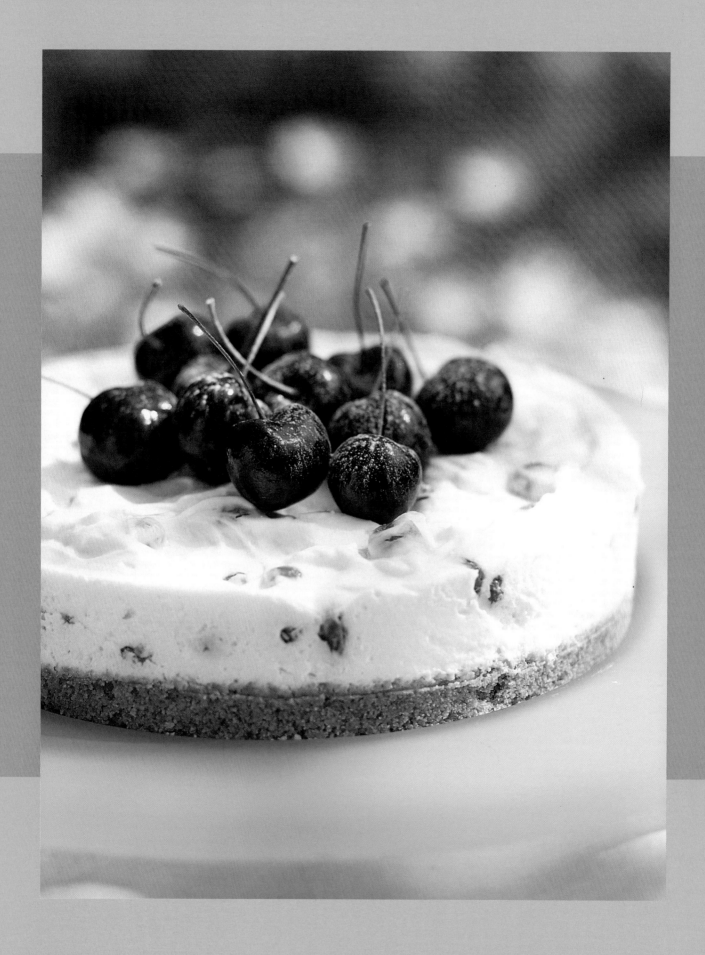

6 Desserts

HOT DESSERTS

COLD DESSERTS

ICED DESSERTS

Raspberry Soufflé Omelet

Here's a deliciously simple dessert with a light, fluffy texture. A hint of almond extract adds an aromatic touch.

2 large eggs at room temperature, separated

2 tablespoons (25 ml) granulated sugar

2–3 drops almond extract

2 teaspoons (10 ml) oil

1 tablespooon (15 ml) warmed pure fruit raspberry jam

8 fresh raspberries, halved, and 2 teaspoons (10 ml) sifted confectioners' sugar, to serve

Serves 2

1   Whisk the egg yolks with the sugar and almond extract until they are light and fluffy.

2   With a clean, dry whisk, whisk the egg whites stiffly in a dry bowl and mix them lightly with the egg yolks and sugar.

3   Preheat the broiler to high. Heat the oil in a non-stick, ovenproof omelet pan, pour in the omelet mixture and cook for about 2–3 minutes until it is just set.

4   Place the omelet beneath the broiler for about a minute until it is browned.

5   Quickly spread with warmed jam, fold over and tip onto a warm plate.

6   Decorate with fresh raspberries and confectioners' sugar and serve immediately.

Baked Bananas with Orange

Baked bananas are naturally sweet, and these are given a refreshing citrus tang with the juice and zest of orange. This is a lovely dessert for winter evenings, as it is both warming and light. Serve it on its own, or with a scoop of low-fat ice cream or frozen yogurt.

4 medium bananas

2 tablespoons (25 ml) unsweetened orange juice

Zest of 1 orange

1 tablespoon (15 ml) dried orange peel

Serves 4

1   Preheat the oven to 425°F (220°C). Make a lengthwise slit in each banana, taking care that the skin doesn't peel off.

2   Cut four square pieces of foil, 12" x 12" (30 cm x 30 cm), and place one banana on each. Pour one-quarter of the juice and zest into each slit.

3   Sprinkle each banana with the dried peel and wrap in a foil parcel, sealing with a double fold on the top and ends, leaving space for steam to expand.

4   Place the foil parcels on a non-stick baking tray and bake in the oven for 15–20 minutes until the bananas are soft.

GRILLED FRUIT KABOBS

Enjoy a mouth-watering feast of tangy grilled fruits coated with a mix of honey and lime juice. In the summer months, you can cook these on an outdoor barbecue. If you're using wooden skewers, remember to soak them in water first. Serve with low-fat plain yogurt.

1   Preheat the broiler and line the tray with foil. Place the fruit in a bowl.

2   Mix the lime juice with the honey and stir into the fruit, making sure that the chunks are coated well on all sides.

3   Thread the chunks of fruit alternately onto four skewers and broil for about 5 minutes until softened.

1 ripe but firm mango, peeled, pitted and cut into bite-sized chunks

½ small pineapple, cored and cut into bite-sized chunks

2 kiwi fruit, peeled and quartered

1 tablespoon (15 ml) lime juice

2 teaspoons (10 ml) liquid honey

Serves 4

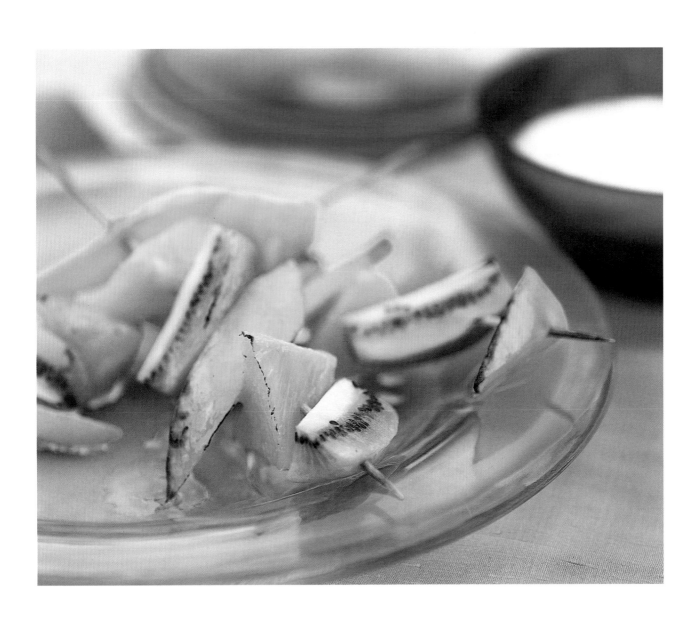

AMARETTO & ALMOND-STUFFED PEACHES

Almond flavors add their intensely aromatic note to the sweet ripeness of peaches in this simple but elegant dish. Peach halves canned in natural juice are an excellent substitute if you don't have fresh ones. The butter is necessary to achieve the right texture, but very little is used, so you can indulge with a clear conscience.

4 very ripe fresh peaches, or 8 peach halves, canned in natural juice and drained

FOR THE STUFFING

⅓ cup (75 ml) ground almonds

1 tablespoon (15 ml) soft butter

2 tablespoons (25 ml) granulated sugar

2 tablespoons (25 ml) Amaretto or other almond liqueur

¼ cup (50 ml) low-fat sour cream or yogurt, to serve

Serves 4

1 Preheat the oven to 375°F (190°C).

2 If you're using canned, drained peaches, go to step 3. If you're using fresh peaches, put them into a bowl of boiling water. Leave for 1 minute, then peel off the skins. Cut through to the pits lengthwise, then twist sharply to separate the two halves. Remove the pits and any fibrous tissue.

3 Mix the almonds with the butter, sugar and liqueur and use this mixture to stuff the peach halves.

4 Arrange the peaches on a lightly greased baking tray, stuffing side up, and bake in the center of the oven for 15 minutes.

5 Serve warm or cold with a swirl of low-fat sour cream or yogurt.

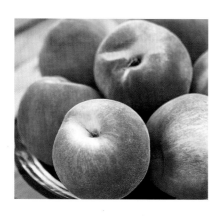

POACHED PEARS WITH FRUIT COULIS

This deceptively simple dessert has an exquisite flavor and needs no added sugar. It tastes particularly delicious if you use a ripe, naturally sweet pear such as Forelle or Red Bartlett. The pears look spectacular if they are left whole—preferably with the stems on, though the poaching time will take about five minutes longer.

4 ripe pears, halved lengthwise and cored

Juice of 1 lemon

FOR THE FRUIT COULIS

8 oz (225 g) mixed unsweetened berries (thawed if frozen)

Sprig of fresh red currants or mint leaves, to decorate

Serves 4

1 Arrange the pears in a large shallow-based pan, with the cored side facing down, in a single layer.

2 Mix the lemon juice with enough cold water to cover the pears. Bring to the boil, lower the heat and simmer gently for 5–10 minutes. The timing depends on the variety and the ripeness of the pears that you use. They should remain quite firm, but soft enough to get a dessert fork through.

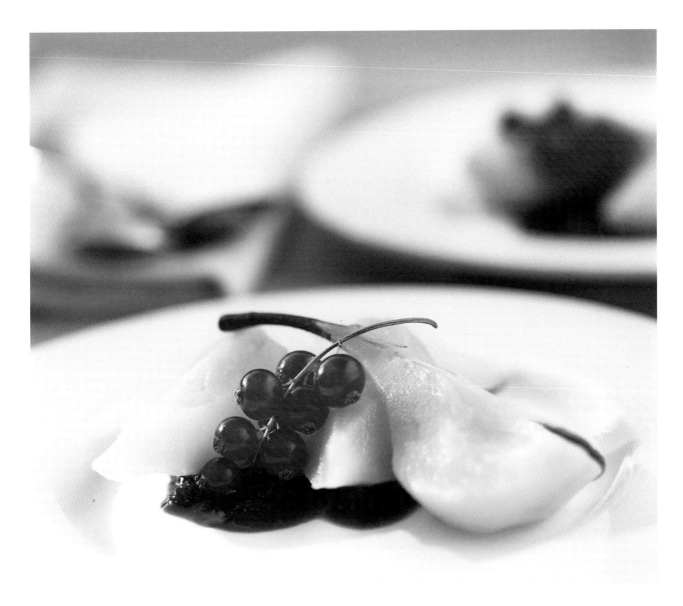

3 Transfer the poached pears to 4 serving plates and leave aside to cool.

4 Meanwhile, make the coulis. Purée the mixed berries in a blender or food processor, then push the mixture through a fine sieve in order to remove the seeds.

5 Spoon or pipe the coulis around the pear halves and decorate with a sprig of fresh red currants or mint leaves before serving.

OLD-FASHIONED BREAD & BUTTER PUDDING

4 slices wholewheat bread

¼ cup (50 ml) whipped or reduced-fat butter

2 tablespoons (25 ml) sugar

⅓ cup (75 ml) raisins

3 medium eggs

1½ cups (375 ml) skim milk

½ teaspoon (2 ml) freshly grated nutmeg

Serves 4

If you have some stale bread, you can use it to make this wonderfully comforting dessert. Any variety of whole-grain bread is fine, although wholewheat gives a lighter result than multigrain.

1 Preheat the oven to 350°F (180°C). Butter each slice of bread with the butter, saving a little to grease the baking dish.

2 Grease a 1-quart (1-liter) baking dish. Cut each slice in half diagonally, leaving the crusts on, and arrange in the dish in alternating layers, each layer sprinkled with the sugar and raisins.

3 Whisk the eggs and milk together, then strain over the bread mixture. Leave to stand for at least 15–20 minutes, until well soaked.

4 Sprinkle with the grated nutmeg and bake for 35–40 minutes until the pudding is puffed up and golden. A knife inserted in the center should come out clean. Serve warm.

APPLE & PLUM CRUMBLE

¾ cup (175 ml) wholewheat flour

1 cup (250 ml) quick-cooking oats

2 tablespoons (25 ml) reduced-fat margarine, chilled and diced

½ cup (125 ml) light brown sugar

5 medium ripe plums, halved and pitted

2 large apples, peeled and sliced

1 teaspoon (5 ml) cinnamon

2 tablespoons (25 ml) water

Serves 4

This is a favorite traditional dessert, and is both wholesome and warming. You can experiment with different combinations of fruit, such as apple and rhubarb or apricot and banana. Serve hot with a low-fat custard or, for a treat, low-fat sour cream .

1 Preheat the oven to 350°F (180°C).

2 Put the flour and oats into a large bowl, add the margarine and rub it in lightly with your fingertips until the mixture resembles coarse crumbs.

3 Stir in half the sugar and mix well.

4 Arrange the plums and apple slices in a lightly greased pie dish. Sprinkle on the remainder of the sugar and the cinnamon, then add the water.

5 Now sprinkle on the crumble mixture, smoothing it over with a fork.

6 Bake above the center of the oven for 35 minutes or until top is golden brown. Serve hot or warm.

Black Forest Crepes

These are delicious made with any variety of jam, but cherry preserves add the authentic Black Forest touch. If crepes are a favorite dessert, it's worth making a double batch and freezing them between sheets of wax paper, ready to be defrosted and filled.

1 Sift the flour and salt into a large bowl. Make a well in the center of the mixture and break in the egg.

2 Add a little milk and beat with a whisk, gradually adding a little more milk at a time, until a smooth batter is formed.

3 Beat for 1–2 more minutes until the surface of the batter is covered with tiny bubbles, then leave to stand for 30 minutes.

4 Brush the base of a non-stick crepe pan with the oil. Heat until sizzling, then pour in one-eighth of the batter, swirling it around to cover the base of the pan.

5 Cook for 1–2 minutes until the underside of the crepe is golden. Using a plastic spatula, loosen the crepe, flip it over, and cook for a further 1–2 minutes. Transfer to a warm plate, and cover with wax paper.

6 Brush the pan with a little more oil and repeat the cooking process for the remainder of the crepes, stacking them between layers of wax paper.

7 When they are ready to serve, spread each crepe with a little of the black cherry preserves (or low-sugar jam) and roll it up.

8 Allow 2 crepes per serving and decorate them with a swirl of low-fat sour cream and a dusting of grated dark chocolate.

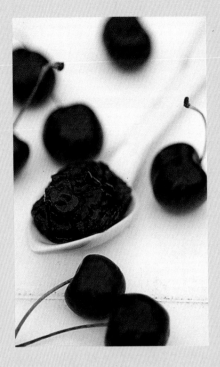

FRESH STRAWBERRY CREPES
For a lower-calorie alternative, pile 1¼ cups (300 ml) fresh strawberry halves and ½ cup (125 ml) Balkan-style yogurt into the crepes instead of the jam and sour cream.

FOR THE CREPES

1 cup (250 ml) all-purpose flour

Pinch of salt

1 large egg

1¼ cups (300 ml) skim milk

2 teaspoons (10 ml) sunflower oil

FOR THE FILLING

⅓ cup (75 ml) low-sugar black cherry preserves, or low-sugar black currant jam

⅓ cup (75 ml) low-fat sour cream and 1 square (1 oz/30 g) dark chocolate, grated, to decorate

Serves 4 (makes 8 crepes)

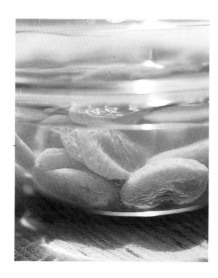

APRICOT & APPLE TARTE TATIN

A tarte tatin is a French classic—an upside-down tart with the pastry baked on top of the fruit, then, after it has been baked, inverted to serve. This recipe uses wholewheat flour and dried apricots, but you can substitute white flour and ready-to-eat apricots if you prefer. Caramelized brown sugar adds a sweet crunch of delicious indulgence.

1   Preheat the oven to 350°F (180°C).

2   To make the pastry, sift the plain and wholewheat flours and the salt into a bowl, adding any bran left behind in the sifter. Cut the margarine into small pieces, and rub it in with your fingertips until the mixture has the texture of fine breadcrumbs. Mix in enough cold water to form a soft dough, then wrap in plastic wrap and chill for 30 minutes.

3   Prepare the upside-down topping. Brush an 8-inch (20-cm) cake pan with half of the sunflower oil. Cut a circle of parchment paper to fit the base, grease it with the remainder of the oil and place it in the base of the pan.

4   Coat the parchment paper with the sugar, pressing it down firmly and evenly.

5   Sprinkle with the cinnamon and arrange the apricots on top, again pressing them down firmly and evenly.

6   Roll out the dough on a lightly floured board and cut out a circle to fit on top of the apricots, pressing down gently. Chill for 15–20 minutes.

7   Bake for 40 minutes or until the pastry is golden.

8   Allow to cool, loosen lightly around the edges with a spatula, and invert the tart onto a large plate. Remove the parchment paper before serving.

FOR THE PASTRY

½ cup (125 ml) all-purpose flour

½ cup (125 ml) wholewheat flour

Pinch of salt

⅓ cup (75 ml) reduced-fat margarine, chilled

2–3 tablespoons (25–45 ml) water

FOR THE TOPPING

2 teaspoons (10 ml) sunflower oil

¾ cup (175 ml) dark brown sugar

1 teaspoon (5 ml) ground cinnamon

1½ cups (375 ml) dried apricots, soaked overnight and drained

Serves 6

CHILLED LEMON & LIME MOUSSE

The clean citrus tang of lemon and lime adds refreshing zest to this classic dessert. You can use lemons or limes on their own, but a combination of the two is spectacular. This mousse does have the richness of whipped cream and sugar, though the cream cheese used is a lower-fat version. It is delicious with Low-sugar Shortbread (see page 117). All in all, a refreshing creamy dessert which has all the freshness of citrus fruits and a touch of Grand Marnier to make it even more special.

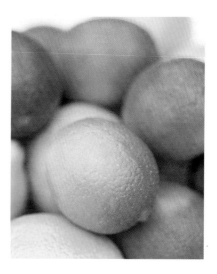

1   Beat the cheese using an electric beater until it is light and fluffy.

2   Add the confectioners' sugar, lemon juice, lime juice and whipped cream and continue to beat until the mixture is soft and creamy.

3   Fold in the Grand Marnier and spoon into individual glasses or dessert dishes.

4   Decorate each dish with mint leaves and the topping of your choice (see below). Chill in the refrigerator.

8 oz (225 g) low-fat cream cheese

¾ cup (175 ml) confectioners' sugar

Juice of 2 lemons

Juice of 2 limes

⅔ cup (150 ml) whipping cream, whipped

1 tablespoon (15 ml) Grand Marnier

Few fresh mint leaves

Serves 4

MOUSSE TOPPINGS

A complementary garnish would be 4 slices each of crystallized lemon and lime, each cut in half. For a fresh fruit alternative, a few seedless grapes or tangerine slices placed on top of each mousse will make an attractive contrast.

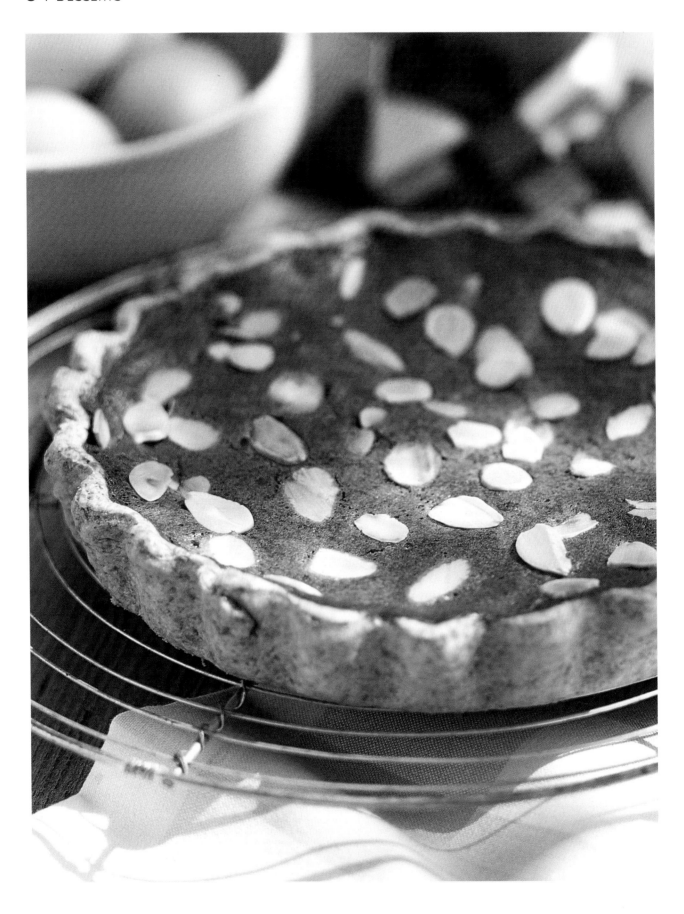

CHOCOLATE & ALMOND CUSTARD TART

This tart is made with an old-fashioned egg custard filling. It is relatively high in fat, so reserve it for special occasions. Always use solid margarine, as the spreadable type is too high in water for successful pastry-making.

1 Preheat the oven to 400°F (200°C). Lightly spray a 9-inch (23-cm) pie pan with cooking spray.

2 Make the pastry in a food processor. Combine the flour, baking powder and salt and process for a few seconds to blend ingredients. Add the chilled margarine or shortening and pulse a few times until the fat is cut into the flour and the pieces are the size of large crumbs.

3 Transfer mixture to a mixing bowl and add just enough of the ice water to moisten the ingredients.

4 Stir together with a fork to bring mixture together into a dough, adding a bit more ice water if mixture remains crumbly. Once it holds together, gather into a ball and press into a disk shape, about 4 inches (10 cm) in diameter.

5 Place the dough between two sheets of wax paper or plastic wap and roll out to about a 12-inch (30-cm) circle. Remove wax paper from the top, wrap the dough over the rolling pin and transfer to the pie pan. Once the pie pan has been lined with pastry, chill it for about 15 minutes.

6 Line the pastry shell with parchment paper or foil and fill with pie weights. Bake for 15–20 minutes or until lightly browned. Remove form the oven, remove the paper or foil and pie weights, and let cool. Reduce oven temperature to 350°F (175°C).

7 Meanwhile, whisk the eggs and sugar together in a bowl until they are light and fluffy.

8 Put the milk, chocolate and vanilla extract into a small saucepan and heat gently, stirring continuously, until the chocolate has completely melted and blended in with the milk. Do not allow the milk to boil.

9 Pour the chocolate mixture into the beaten eggs, mix well, then pour into the pastry and top with the flaked almonds. Bake for 30–40 minutes until the pastry is golden and the custard has just set.

10 Cool on a wire rack before serving.

FOR THE PASTRY

1⅓ cups (325 ml) all-purpose flour

½ teaspoon (2 ml) baking powder

¼ teaspoon (1 ml) salt

6 tablespoons (90 ml) regular margarine or vegetable shortening, chilled, cut into small pieces

3–4 tablespoons (45–50 ml) ice water

Cooking spray

FOR THE FILLING

2 medium eggs, lightly beaten

2 tablespoons (25 ml) granulated sugar

1 cup less 2 tablespoons (225 ml) skim milk

2 squares (2 oz/60 g) good quality dark chocolate (75% cocoa solids), broken into small pieces

2–3 drops pure vanilla extract

2 tablespoons (25 ml) flaked almonds, to decorate

Serves 8

CINNAMON CUSTARD TART

Omit the chocolate and make the egg custard as above. Add 1 level teaspoon (5 ml) of cinnamon, the zest of half a lemon, a few drops of vanilla extract and some grated nutmeg. Dust with cinnamon before serving.

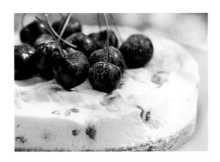

Lemon & Raisin Cheesecake with Cherries

Cheesecake is generally high in fat and calories when made with full-fat cream cheese. But you can go ahead and enjoy this feather-light version, as the filling is virtually fat-free. For a spectacular topping, use very ripe cherries. (For this recipe you can use soft margarine, since you are not making pastry.)

1 Mix the graham crackers thoroughly with the margarine. Press firmly into the base of an 8-inch (20-cm) loose-bottomed cake pan and chill for 1 hour or until firm.

2 Follow package directions for dissolving gelatin, then put the dissolved gelatin into a blender or food processor along with the lemon juice, cheese, yogurt and sugar.

3 Blend for a few seconds and transfer to a large bowl. Mix in the raisins.

4 Pour onto the crumb base and chill. After about 2 hours, or when just beginning to firm up, place the confectioners' sugar in a little sifter and shake over the cherries. Place the sugared cherries on top of the cake.

5 Return to the refrigerator and chill until completely set.

FOR THE BASE

2 cups (500 ml) crushed graham crackers

⅓ cup (75 ml) reduced-fat margarine, very soft

FOR THE FILLING

2 envelopes gelatin

Juice of 1 lemon

1⅓ cups (325 ml) low-fat ricotta cheese

⅔ cup (150 ml) low-fat (1–2% M.F.) plain yogurt

¼ cup (50 ml) granulated sugar

⅓ cup (75 ml) raisins

¾ cup (175 ml) very ripe cherries

2 teaspoons (10 ml) confectioners' sugar

Serves 8

Petits Coeurs à la Crème

Traditionally this classic French dessert is made in small, perforated heart-shaped molds—hence the name "petits coeurs." You can get the molds from specialist kitchenware suppliers, but alternatively, you can use one large colander or sieve. The recipe benefits from being lower in fat and sugar than the classic version, as low-fat ricotta cheese and low-fat yogurt replace the traditionally richer ingredients.

1 Process the cheese, yogurt and milk in a blender or food processor until smooth, then transfer to a mixing bowl.

2 Add the extract and sugar and mix thoroughly.

8 oz (250 g) low-fat ricotta cheese

⅓ cup (75 ml) low-fat (1–2% M.F.) plain yogurt

2 tablespoons (25 ml) skim milk

1 teaspoon (5 ml) vanilla or almond extract

¼ cup (50 ml) granulated sugar

1½ cups (375 ml) strawberries

4 small sprigs mint leaves

Serves 4

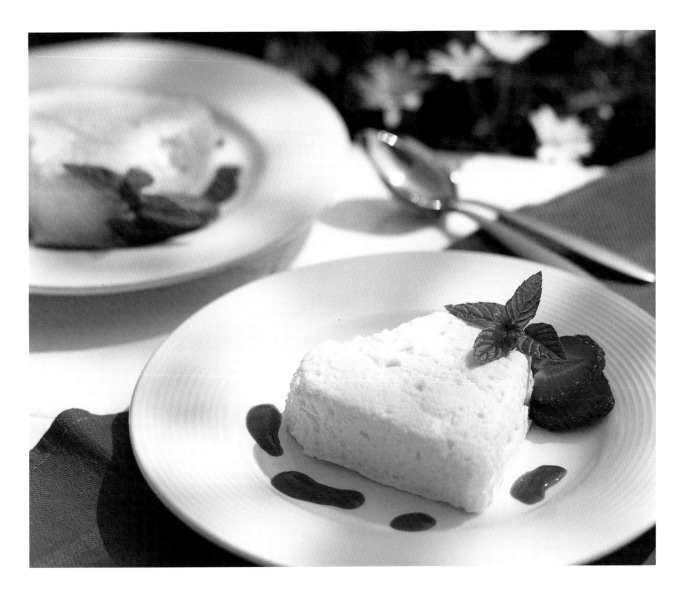

3   Spoon into 4 small perforated molds or 1 large one (see introduction
    above), lined with damp cheesecloth and carefully smooth the tops.

4   Stand molds on a wire rack over a baking tray and leave to drain for 6–8
    hours in the refrigerator.

5   Meanwhile, purée the berries in a blender or food processor, reserving 4
    berries, halved, for the garnish.

6   To serve, turn out and encircle with the puréed berries. Garnish with fresh
    mint sprigs and the reserved berries.

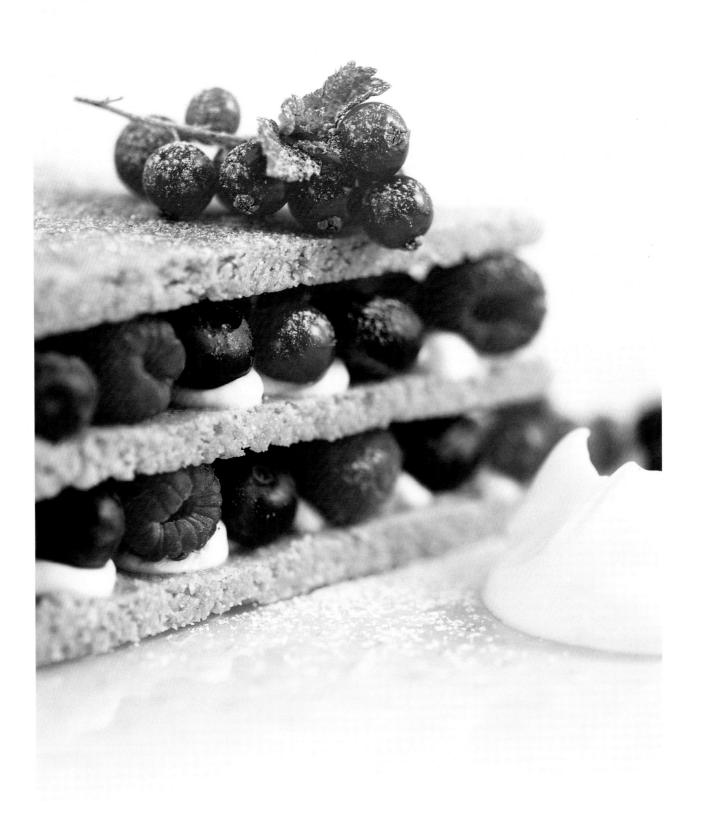

RASPBERRY & BLUEBERRY SHORTBREAD STACKS

These shortbread treats are simple to make and surprisingly rich, despite the sneaky low-fat sour cream. The shortbread is crunchy and crumbly—make sure you work the mixture well into the corners of the pan, making the surface as even as possible, and mark out the divisions deeply before baking.

1 Preheat the oven to 300°F (150°C). Lightly grease and line an 8-inch (20-cm) square cake pan with parchment paper.

2 Cream the butter and sugar together until light and fluffy.

3 Sift in the flour and add the rice flour, a little at a time, mixing steadily with a wooden spoon. Use your fingers to make a smooth but firm dough.

4 Press gently into the prepared pan, making sure you distribute the mixture evenly and flatly. Cut all the way through into 12 squares.

5 Bake for 50 or 55 minutes, or until the shortbread is firm and lightly browned. Let cool slightly. Remove from the pan, gently break into 12 pieces and allow to cool.

6 When you are ready to serve, top four of the shortbread squares with half the berries and half the sour cream.

7 Add four more squares on top and then add a layer of the remaining berries and sour cream.

8 Finally, lay the last four squares on top, and decorate with a sprig of red currants or fresh mint. Sift the confectioners' sugar and sprinkle about a teaspoon (5 ml) onto each stack.

FOR THE SHORTBREAD

⅓ cup plus 2 tablespoons (100 ml) butter

3 tablespoons (45 ml) granulated sugar

¾ cup (175 ml) all-purpose flour

½ cup (125 ml) rice flour

FOR THE FILLING

½ cup (125 ml) fresh raspberries

¾ cup (175 ml) fresh blueberries

¼ cup (50 ml) low-fat sour cream

FOR THE TOPPING

Sprig of red currants or fresh mint

4 teaspoons (20 ml) confectioners' sugar

Serves 4

Raspberry & Ginger Sundaes

This is such an easy dessert to make, yet it tastes really good. Spicy stem ginger (available in Asian markets), sweet raspberries and sour cream make a gratifying blend of flavors and contrasting textures.

FOR THE COOKIE BASE

2 cups (500 ml) low-fat ginger cookies, crushed

⅓ cup (75 ml) reduced-fat margarine, melted

FOR THE TOPPING

½ cup (125 ml) low-fat sour cream

2 small pieces stem ginger, finely chopped

3 tablespoons (45 ml) granulated sugar

2½ cups (625 ml) fresh raspberries

Serves 4

1 Mix the crushed cookies with the reduced-fat margarine and spoon into 4 individual dessert or sundae dishes. Chill for 30 minutes, or until firm.

2 Mix the sour cream with the chopped ginger and about half the sugar, then spoon it over each crushed cookie base.

3 Top with the raspberries, sprinkle with the remaining sugar, and chill again before serving.

Exotic Fruit Salad with Cardamom

This luscious salad is made from an exotic mix of fruits scented with cardamom. You can use any combination of fruit you like, but the secret is to have a variety of colors and textures. Serve with a final swirl of low-fat sour cream for creamy contrast.

FOR THE SYRUP

¼ cup (50 ml) granulated sugar

Zest of 1 lemon

8 green cardamom pods, cracked slightly, but still retaining their seeds

1¼ cups (300 ml) water

2 large mangoes, skin and pit removed and cut into cubes

2 bananas, peeled and sliced

2 papayas, peeled and diced

1 large red apple, cut into quarters, core removed and sliced (leave skin on)

2 small red pears, prepared in the same way as the apple above

Serves 6–8

1 First make the syrup. Place the sugar in a saucepan with the lemon zest and cardamom. Add the water and heat until boiling, then lower the heat and simmer for 2 minutes.

2 Remove from the heat, add a couple of ice cubes to cool the syrup, then pour it into a large bowl.

3 As you prepare the fruit, add it to the syrup immediately, and mix together well. Otherwise the fruit will go brown with exposure to the air.

4 Cover and place in the refrigerator for at least 1 hour before serving so that the flavors have time to mingle.

5 Remove the cardamom pods before you serve (the seeds are edible).

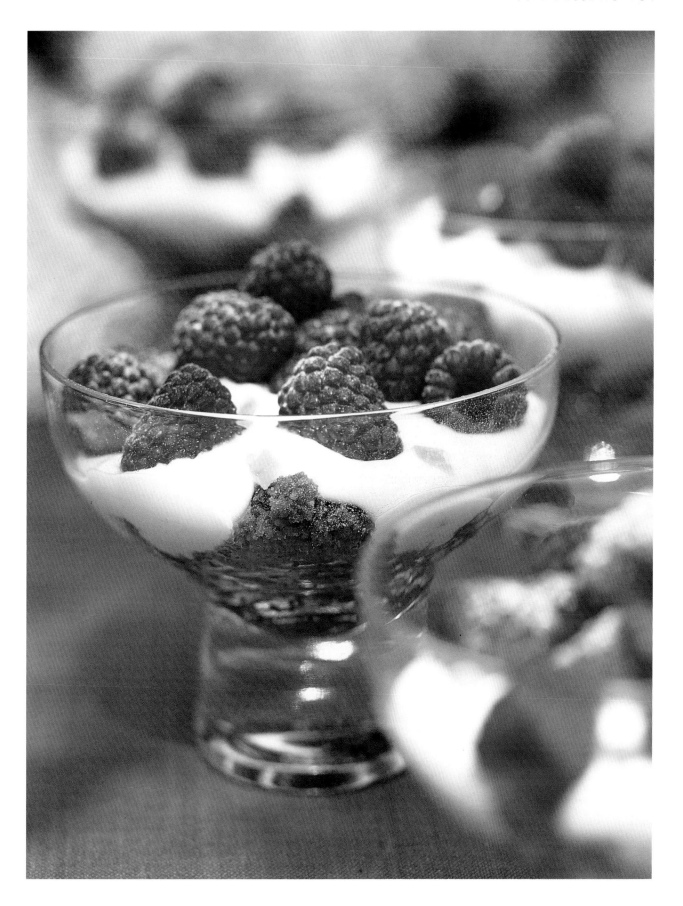

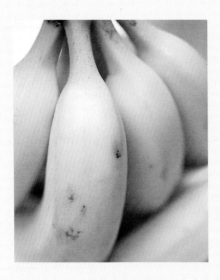

FOR THE ICE CREAM

3 large ripe bananas, peeled
and coarsely chopped

Juice of 1 lemon

1¼ cups (300 ml) can low-fat evaporated
milk, chilled

1 tablespoon (15 ml) sugar

FOR THE TOPPING

3 squares (3 oz/90 g) dark chocolate

2 tablespoons (25 ml) water

4 teaspoons (20 ml) reduced-fat
margarine

⅓ cup (75 ml) hazelnuts, coarsely
chopped

Serves 4

BANANA ICE CREAM WITH CHOCOLATE & HAZELNUT TOPPING

This homemade ice cream is a special treat, mingling the sweet flavors of bananas and chocolate with the satisfying crunch of hazelnuts. Serve this dessert after a high-fiber main meal, to slow down the absorption of its sugar.

1 Place a 1-quart (1-liter) plastic container (with lid) in the freezer to chill. Mash the bananas in a large bowl until thick and pulpy. Add the lemon juice and mash again.

2 In a separate bowl, whip the evaporated milk with an electric beater until it is thick and frothy and almost doubled in volume.

3 Add this to the mashed bananas, a little at a time, beating continuously until it is thick and smooth. Stir in the sugar.

4 Pour into the pre-chilled container, cover and freeze for 1 hour or until just beginning to set around the edges.

5 Remove from freezer and whisk thoroughly until smooth, re-cover and freeze again for 2–3 hours, checking after two hours, until frozen through.

6 Meanwhile, make the topping. Cut the chocolate into pieces and put them into a small pan with the water. Place over a larger pan of gently simmering water and stir until completely melted. Remove from the heat and beat in the margarine. Allow to cool, and stir in the chopped hazelnuts.

7 If the ice cream is frozen solid, move it to the main body of the refrigerator for 30 minutes before serving, to soften slightly. Pour the chocolate sauce over the ice cream just before serving.

SUMMER BERRY FROZEN DESSERT

You can use any mixture of summer berries for this, but it's a good idea to include blueberries or blackberries, as they give a gloriously rich color. You can also use frozen fruits, but make sure they are thawed and drained before blending.

1 Place a 1-quart (1-liter) plastic container (with lid) in the freezer to chill. Put the fruit into a blender or food processor with the sugar and blend for about 1 minute until it is puréed.

2 Rub the purée through a sieve to remove any seeds, then mix in the lemon juice and yogurt.

3 Pour the mixture into the pre-chilled container, cover and freeze for 1 hour until it is semi-solid.

4 Remove from the freezer and beat the mixture until it is smooth and creamy. Cover and freeze again for 3 hours, checking after 2 hours, until frozen solid.

5 Move the dessert to the refrigerator 30 minutes before serving, and decorate it with the whole raspberries.

1 cup (250 ml) of raspberries, 2 cups (500 ml) of strawberries, and 1 cup (250 ml) of blueberries or blackberries

¼ cup (50 ml) granulated sugar

1 teaspoon (5 ml) lemon juice

1¼ cups (300 ml) low-fat (1–2% M.F.) plain yogurt

¼ cup (50 ml) fresh raspberries, to decorate

Serves 4

STRAWBERRY & MASCARPONE SORBET

This sorbet is a particularly refreshing summer dessert. Though sorbets can be a time-consuming dessert to make, the delicious combination of the creamy Italian cheese and the fresh strawberries make the extra effort worthwhile.

1 Place a 1-quart (1-liter) plastic container (with lid) in the freezer to chill. Put the strawberries into a food processor or blender, and blend with the sugar and lemon juice for about 1 minute.

2 Beat the mascarpone cheese with the yogurt, then mix in the strawberry purée. Spoon the mixture into the pre-chilled container. Cover and freeze for about 1 hour until crystals start to form around the edges.

3 Remove from the freezer and whisk briskly. Return to the freezer and repeat this stage 2 or 3 times until the sorbet is smooth and completely frozen solid.

4 Scoop into long-stemmed glasses and serve garnished with strawberries and fresh mint.

2 cups (500 ml) fresh strawberries, hulled

⅓ cup (75 ml) granulated sugar

1 tablespoon (15 ml) lemon juice

⅔ cup (150 ml) mascarpone cheese

⅔ cup (150 ml) Balkan-style yogurt

fresh strawberries and fresh mint leaves, to serve

Serves 4

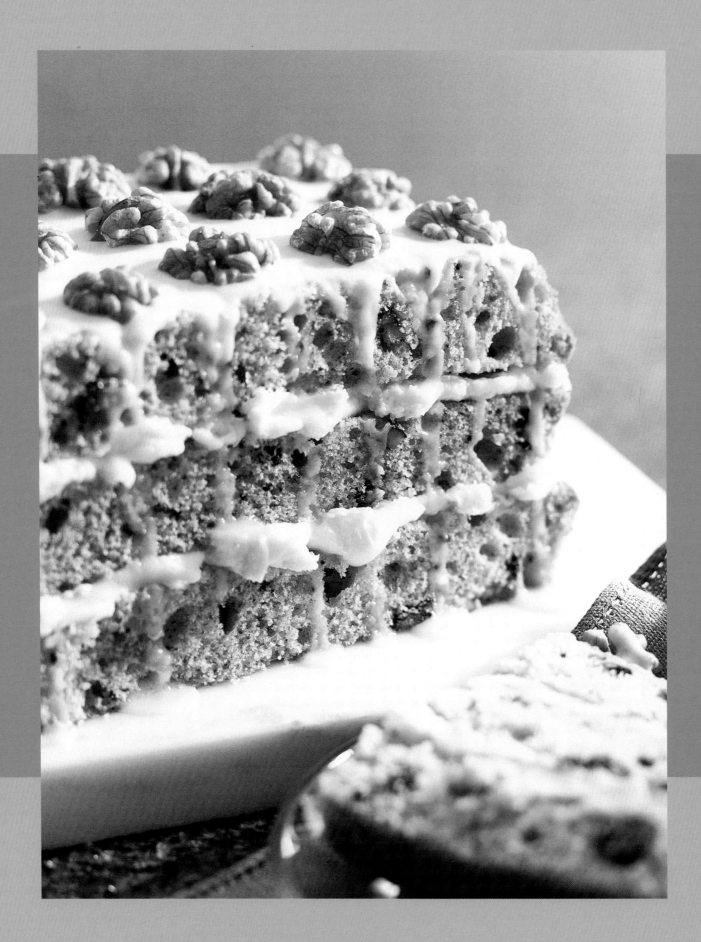

7

Cakes, Cookies & Breads

FRUIT SCONES

1 cup (250 ml) all-purpose white flour

1 cup (250 ml) wholewheat flour

2¼ teaspoons (10 ml) baking powder

Pinch of salt

¼ cup (50 ml) soft margarine (at room temperature)

2 tablespoons (25 ml) granulated sugar

⅓ cup (75 ml) raisins

⅔ cup (150 ml) skim milk (keep 2 teaspoons (10 ml) aside for brushing the tops of the scones before baking)

Makes 18

Freshly made scones are a real treat—and these are so easy to make. Serve them simply with margarine, or indulge yourself and smother them in low-fat cream cheese, fresh strawberries and a sprinkling of chopped nuts or flaked chocolate. You could use all white flour or all wholewheat, but the 50/50 mixture used here works well and provides a healthy balance without being too heavy.

1 Preheat the oven to 425°F (220°C). Sift the flours into a bowl with the baking powder and salt, tipping any leftover bran into the sifted mixture.

2 Lightly rub in the margarine with your fingertips until the mixture has the consistency of fine bread crumbs.

3 Mix in the sugar and raisins (the same quantities of dried mixed peel can be used instead) and add the milk a little at a time, mixing well until a soft dough is formed.

4 Turn out onto a lightly floured board and roll out to a thickness of ¾ inch (2 cm). Using a 1½-inch (4-cm) pastry cutter, cut out the scones, re-rolling the leftover dough as necessary until you have used it all.

5 Place the scones on a lightly greased baking sheet, brush the tops with a little skim milk to glaze, and bake near the top of the oven for 15–20 minutes until golden.

6 Cool on a wire rack until the scones are just warm, then serve.

GRANDMA'S HOMEMADE GINGERBREAD

This old-fashioned cake fills the kitchen with delicious spicy aromas while it is baking. As this gingerbread won't keep well for more than 2–3 days, you might want to freeze some for later.

1 Preheat the oven to 350°F (180°C).

2 Lightly grease a square, shallow 8-inch (20-cm) cake pan and line it with parchment paper.

3 Sift the flour and baking soda and mix with the sugar, cinnamon, ginger and raisins.

4 In a large bowl, cream the margarine with the molasses, then mix in the flour and raisin mixture.

5 Add the beaten egg and milk, mixing thoroughly to a fairly stiff consistency.

6 Spoon the mixture into the greased and lined pan and bake for 25 minutes.

7 Reduce the oven temperature to 300°F (170°C), and continue baking for 25–35 minutes, or until a skewer inserted into the center comes out clean.

8 Cool in the pan for 15 minutes, then turn out and leave to cool completely on a wire rack. Cut into 16 squares before serving.

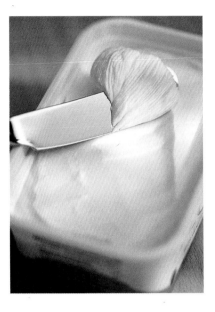

2½ cups (625 ml) all-purpose flour

1 teaspoon (5 ml) baking soda

Pinch of salt

½ cup (125 ml) dark brown sugar

2 teaspoons (10 ml) ground cinnamon

2 teaspoons (10 ml) ground ginger

1 cup (250 ml) raisins

½ cup (125 ml) reduced-fat margarine at room temperature

¼ cup (50 ml) molasses

1 large egg, beaten

⅔ cup (150 ml) skim milk, just warm

Makes 16 slices

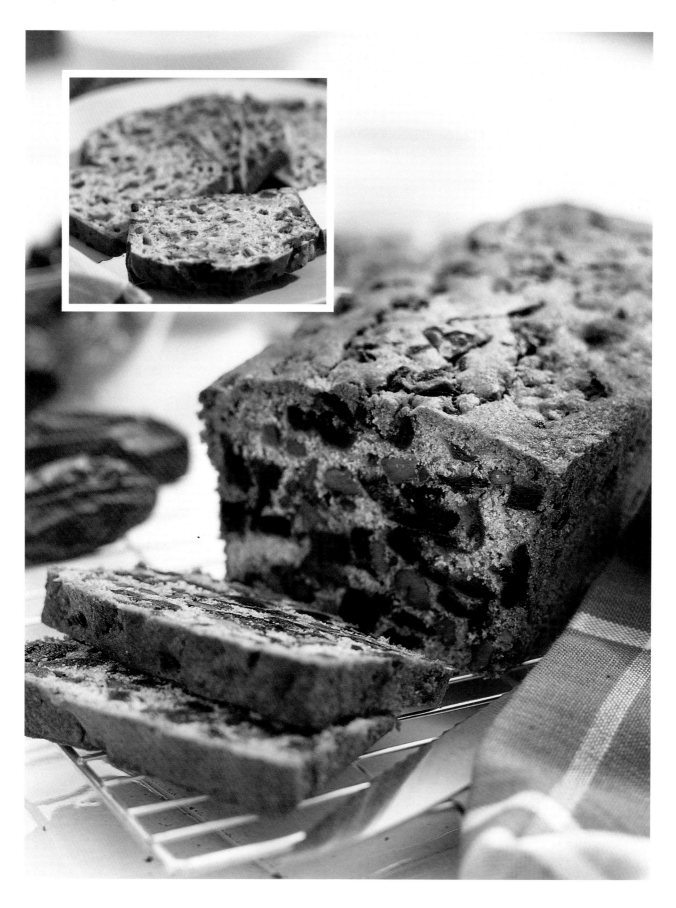

DATE & BANANA LOAF

This is a sumptuously spicy, moist fruit loaf that contains no extra fat or sugar, and relies completely on the natural sugar content of the fruits for its sweetness. Try it for yourself—it's very easy to make.

1   Preheat the oven to 350°F (180°C).

2   Lightly grease and line an 8 x 4 inch (1.5 liter) loaf pan with parchment paper.

3   Put the chopped dates, bananas, egg and milk into a blender or food processor and process for a minute or two until the mixture is smooth.

4   Sift the flour, salt, cinnamon and ginger into a mixing bowl, then add the fruit mixture and stir by hand until thoroughly blended.

5   Turn the mixture into the prepared pan and bake in the center of the oven for about 30 minutes. If the loaf is fairly brown on the top, turn the heat down to 325°F (170°C). If not, leave it as it is, and bake for a further 25–30 minutes, or until a skewer inserted into the center comes out clean.

6   Leave the loaf to cool in the pan for 10 minutes, then turn it out and leave it to cool completely on a wire rack.

1 cup (250 ml) pitted dates, coarsely chopped

2 cups (500 ml) ripe bananas, peeled and coarsely chopped

1 large egg

½ cup (125 ml) skim milk

1¾ cups (425 ml) self-rising flour

Pinch of salt

½ teaspoon (2 ml) ground cinnamon

½ teaspoon (2 ml) ground ginger

Makes 15 slices

FRUIT & WALNUT LOAF

Walnuts add their own rich flavor and texture to this satisfyingly rich loaf, while the fruits contribute their own sweetness and moisture. It's also low in sugar and high in fiber, making this an excellent healthy choice for people with diabetes.

1   Preheat the oven to 350°F (180°C).

2   Cream the butter and sugar together and mix in the beaten egg.

3   Mix in the flours and baking powder, and stir in the milk until the mixture has a thick consistency.

4   Add the fruit and nuts and mix well.

5   Spoon the mixture into an 8 x 4 inch (1.5 liter) greased loaf pan and bake for 1 hour (test to ensure that it is fully cooked by inserting a skewer and checking that it comes out clean).

6   Cool the loaf on a wire rack before slicing.

⅓ cup (75 ml) butter

⅔ cup (150 ml) granulated sugar

1 large egg, beaten

1 cup (250 ml) all-purpose flour

1 cup (250 ml) wholewheat flour

2 teaspoons (10 ml) baking powder

¾ cup (175 ml) skim milk

1¼ cups (300 ml) dates, pitted and chopped

1¼ cups (300 ml) prunes, pitted and chopped into small pieces

1¼ cups (300 ml) walnut pieces, roughly chopped

Makes 18–20 pieces

QUICK & EASY SWISS ROLL

This feather-light sponge cake takes just minutes to bake and is quite simple to prepare. The only tricky part is rolling it up, so follow the instructions carefully. If the edges seem a little crisp after baking, it's a good idea to trim them before rolling or the sponge may crack.
Any flavor of reduced-sugar jam may be used.

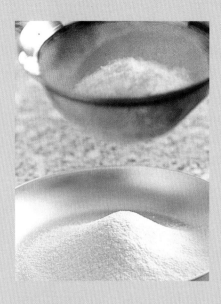

¾ cup (175 ml) all-purpose flour, sifted

Pinch of salt

1 teaspoon (5 ml) baking powder

3 medium eggs

⅓ cup, plus 2 tablespoons (100 ml) granulated sugar

1 teaspoon (5 ml) pure vanilla extract

1 tablespoon (15 ml) confectioners' sugar

3 tablespoons (45 ml) reduced-sugar raspberry jam, to fill

Makes 8 slices

1   Preheat the oven to 425°F (220°C).

2   Lightly grease and line a jell-roll pan with parchment paper.

3   Sift the flour, salt and baking powder into a bowl.

4   In another larger bowl placed over a pan of hot water, whisk the eggs and sugar with an electric beater until they are thick and creamy.

5   Add the vanilla extract and lightly fold in the flour mixture, using a large metal spoon.

6   Tip the batter into the prepared pan, spreading it out evenly to the corners and bake for 6–8 minutes. Remove it from the oven when it feels springy to the touch.

7   Place a sheet of parchment paper on top of a clean dish towel and sprinkle the paper with the confectioners' sugar. Turn the sponge cake out onto the parchment paper, crust side down, and remove the paper.

8   About 1 inch (2½ cm) from one of the long edges, make a shallow cut halfway through the sponge cake. Fold this "cut" section over onto the rest of the sponge—this is the first "roll."

9   Continue by using the parchment paper to carefully roll up the rest of the sponge cake.

10 Leave the roll to cool on a wire rack and when it is cold carefully unroll it and spread with the jam about ½ inch (1 cm) from the edges.

11 Roll it up again carefully and slice before serving.

WALNUT LAYER CAKE

This light, low-fat mixture makes a delicate, melt-in-the-mouth cake. It's versatile too—you can serve it for an informal treat, but it would also be perfect for a birthday cake. You can vary the filling and topping as the mood takes you.

1 Preheat the oven to 325°F (170°C).

2 Lightly grease and line a jelly-roll pan with parchment paper.

3 Sift the flour, salt and baking powder into a bowl.

4 Cream the margarine and sugar together until light and fluffy, then beat in the almond extract.

5 Add the beaten eggs, a little at a time, beating well after each addition. Add a little of the flour mixture if there is any sign of curdling.

6 Now add the remaining flour mixture, a little at a time, gently but thoroughly folding it in with a large spoon. Add the milk to give a smooth consistency, and stir in the chopped walnuts.

7 Turn the mixture into the prepared pan, smoothing it evenly into the corners, and bake for 25 minutes. A skewer inserted in the center should come out clean. If it's at all sticky, turn the oven down to 300°F (150°C) and bake for a further 10 minutes.

8 Cool in the pan for 15 minutes, then very gently remove from the pan, peel off the paper and leave on a wire rack until completely cold.

9 Cut horizontally into 3 rectangular cakes, to use as 3 layers, trimming the tops of 2 of them, if necessary, to provide flat surfaces.

10 To make the filling, mix the low-fat cream cheese and the confectioners' sugar and spread over 2 of the layers.

11 Top with the third layer of cake and cover it with the topping (dip the blade of a knife in hot water to give the topping a smooth and even surface). Decorate with the walnut halves.

RASPBERRY LAYER CAKE

Follow steps 1–9, using vanilla extract instead of almond and omitting the walnuts. To make the filling, mix 4 oz (115 g) low-fat cream cheese with 3 tablespoons (45 ml) reduced-sugar raspberry jam and spread over 2 layers. Add the top layer, ice it as above, and decorate with 2 tablespoons (25 ml) chopped candied cherries.

2 cups (500 ml) all-purpose flour

Pinch of salt

2 teaspoons (10 ml) baking powder

½ cup (125 ml) reduced-fat margarine, at room temperature

½ cup (125 ml) granulated sugar

1 teaspoon (5 ml) almond extract

2 large eggs, beaten

½ cup (125 ml) low-fat milk

⅔ cup (150 ml) chopped walnuts

FOR THE FILLING

4 oz (115 g) low-fat cream cheese

2 tablespoons (25 ml) confectioners' sugar

FOR THE TOPPING

⅓ cup (75 ml) sifted confectioners' sugar, mixed with 2½ teaspoons (12 ml) warm water

⅔ cup (150 ml) walnut halves, to decorate

Makes 12 pieces

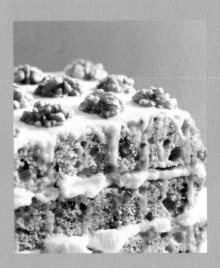

Carrot Cake

This moist carrot cake has a delicious flavor. You can also use the cream cheese as icing and sprinkle some chopped nuts. Or, if you prefer, simply omit the cheese altogether.

1¼ cups (300 ml) wholewheat flour

Pinch of salt

2½ teaspoons (12 ml) baking powder

1 teaspoon (5 ml) ground cinnamon

1 teaspoon (5 ml) ground ginger

½ cup (125 ml) light brown sugar

¾ cup (175 ml) raisins, soaked overnight in ½ cup (125 ml) unsweetened orange juice

4 medium carrots, peeled and finely grated

1 tablespoon (15 ml) sunflower oil

2 medium egg whites, at room temperature

3½ oz (100 g) low-fat cream cheese beaten with 2 teaspoons (10 ml) sifted confectioners' sugar

Makes 12 slices

1   Preheat the oven to 325°F (170°C). Lightly grease an 8 x 4 inch (1.5 liter) loaf pan and line it with parchment paper.

2   Sift the flour, salt, baking powder, cinnamon and ginger into a large bowl, tipping in any bran left in the sifter.

3   Stir in the sugar, raisins with their juice, carrots and oil and mix well.

4   Beat the egg whites until they stand up in soft peaks, then fold lightly but thoroughly into the carrot mixture, using a large spoon or spatula.

5   Pour into the pan and bake in the center of the oven for about 1¼ hours, or until a skewer inserted in the center of the cake comes out clean.

6   Cool in the pan for 10 minutes, then turn out onto a wire rack and peel off the lining paper. When completely cool, cut in half horizontally and fill with the sweetened cream cheese.

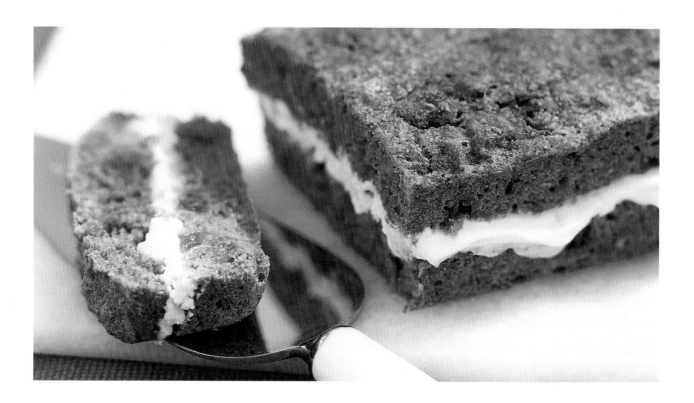

ORANGE & ALMOND CAKE

Next time you decide to make freshly squeezed orange juice, don't throw away the fruit "shells." Grate the zest finely and use it in this Portuguese treat. Traditionally the ratio of flour and almonds is half and half, but this version gives a much lighter texture.

1 Preheat the oven to 350°F (180°C).

2 Lightly grease the base of an 8-inch (20-cm) non-stick baking pan and line with parchment paper.

3 Sift the flour, salt and baking powder together.

4 Beat the eggs until they are light and frothy.

5 Beat the margarine and sugar together until smooth and creamy. Add the beaten eggs gradually, beating well between each addition. If the mixture shows any signs of curdling, beat in a little of the flour mixture.

6 Stir in the flour mixture together with the ground almonds, almond extract and orange zest and mix lightly to a thick, fluid (but not runny) consistency, adding a little orange juice or water if necessary.

7 Pour into the prepared pan, smooth the top, and bake in the center of the oven for about 45–50 minutes, or until a skewer comes out clean when inserted into the center.

8 Strip off the parchment paper and leave the cake to cool on a wire rack.

¾ cup (175 ml) all-purpose flour

Pinch of salt

2 teaspoons (10 ml) baking powder

2 large eggs

½ cup (125 ml) reduced-fat margarine, at room temperature

⅓ cup plus 2 tablespoons (100 ml) granulated sugar

⅓ cup (75 ml) ground almonds

½ teaspoon (2 ml) almond extract

2 teaspoons (10 ml) finely grated orange zest

Makes 10 slices

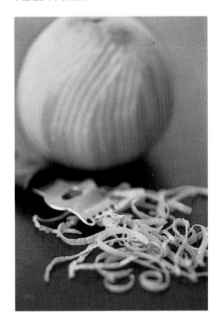

Rich Fruit Cake

2 cups (500 ml) dried mixed fruit (dried figs, apricots, dates, raisins, etc.), finely chopped together

⅔ cup (150 ml) dry cider or unsweetened apple juice

½ cup (125 ml) candied cherries, chopped

⅓ cup (75 ml) chopped walnuts or pecans

1 cup (250 ml) all-purpose flour

1 cup (250 ml) wholewheat flour

2 teaspoons (10 ml) baking powder

1 teaspoon (5 ml) ground cinnamon

½ teaspoon (2 ml) ground nutmeg

½ teaspoon (2 ml) ground cloves

½ cup (125 ml) sunflower oil

3 medium eggs

¾ cup (175 ml) brown sugar

2 teaspoons (10 ml) brandy or rum

Maturing time: 3 days–4 weeks

Makes 20 slices

Here's a cake that's rich, fruity and full of goodness. Because it's made with sunflower oil rather than butter, it's low in saturated fat, and both the fruit and nuts are packed with valuable fiber. It is ideal for icing and decorating on special occasions such as Christmas, birthdays and anniversaries.

1   Soak the mixed fruit overnight in the cider or apple juice, then mix in the cherries and nuts.

2   Preheat the oven to 325°F (170°C). Lightly grease and line an 8-inch (20-cm) cake pan with parchment paper.

3   Sift the flours with the baking powder and ground spices, emptying any leftover bran into the bowl.

4   In a large bowl, beat the sunflower oil with the eggs and sugar. Add the brandy or rum, fruit, nuts and cider or juice, and mix thoroughly.

5   Fold the dry ingredients, a bit at a time, into the egg and fruit mixture, using a large metal spoon and mixing all the time until smooth.

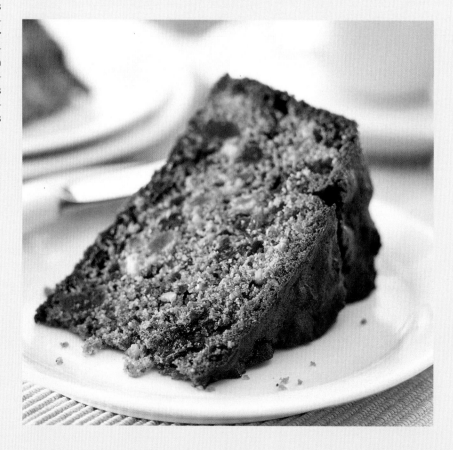

6   Transfer the mixture into the prepared pan and bake for 1 hour 20 minutes
    or until a skewer inserted in the center comes out clean. If the top gets too
    brown, cover it with a double layer of parchment paper.

7   Allow to cool in the pan for about 1 hour, then transfer to a wire rack.
    When cold, wrap in plastic wrap or aluminum foil and store in an airtight
    container for at least 3 days before serving.

MINCEMEAT TARTS

*These mouth-watering tarts are relatively low in fat and sugar, yet
they are still moist and full of festive flavor. This homemade mincemeat
is fragrant with added cinnamon, brandy and ginger. The recipe
makes enough mincemeat for 2 batches of tarts. Meanwhile, it will
keep for a week in a screw-top jar in the refrigerator. For the pastry,
be sure to use solid margarine.*

1   Make the mincemeat. Soak the mixed fruit and grated apple in the cinna-
    mon, margarine, ginger, orange juice, and the rum or brandy overnight.

2   Make the pastry in a food processor. Combine the flour, baking powder
    and salt and process for a few seconds to blend ingredients. Add the
    chilled margarine or shortening and pulse a few times until the fat is cut
    into the flour and the pieces are the size of large crumbs.

3   Transfer the mixture to a mixing bowl and add just enough of the ice water
    to moisten the ingredients.

4   Stir together with a fork to bring mixture together into a dough, adding
    a bit more ice water if mixture remains crumbly. Once it holds together,
    gather together into a ball and press into a disk shape, about 4 inches
    (10 cm) in diameter.

5   Put the pastry into a plastic bag or wrap in plastic wrap and chill in the
    refrigerator for 30 minutes.

6   Preheat the oven to 400°F (200°C), and lightly spray a muffin tin with
    cooking spray. Roll out half of the pastry and, using a 2½-inch (6-cm)
    pastry cutter, cut out 12 circles to line the prepared tin.

7   Spoon one-half of the mincemeat into the prepared pastry shells.

8   Roll out the remainder of the pastry to make lids for the tarts. Dampen the
    edges of the pastry in the tin and cover each tart with a pastry lid, pressing
    the edges together gently but firmly to seal.

9   Brush the tops of the tarts lightly with milk and bake for 15–20 minutes
    until crisp and golden.

FOR THE MINCEMEAT

¾ cup (175 ml) dried mixed fruit (see previous recipe)

1 dessert apple, peeled and grated

1 teaspoon (5 ml) each ground cinnamon and ground ginger

2 tablespoons (25 ml) reduced-fat margarine

⅓ cup (75 ml) unsweetened orange juice

½ teaspoon (2 ml) rum or brandy

FOR THE PASTRY

1⅓ cups (325 ml) all-purpose flour

½ teaspoon (2 ml) baking powder

¼ teaspoon (1 ml) salt

6 tablespoons (90 ml) regular margarine or vegetable shortening, chilled, cut into small pieces

3–4 tablespoons (45–50 ml) ice water

Cooking spray

2 teaspoons (10 ml) skim milk, to glaze

PEANUT BUTTER & WHITE CHOCOLATE COOKIES

A well-stocked cookie jar is sure to be popular with everyone in the family—especially when you fill it with these crunchy treats. Commercially made cookies often contain additives to make them last longer. It makes sense to bake your own, so you know exactly what you're eating.

1¾ cups (425 ml) all-purpose flour

½ teaspoon (2 ml) baking powder

½ cup (125 ml) reduced-fat margarine

⅓ cup (75 ml) granulated sugar

⅓ cup (75 ml) natural chunky peanut butter

⅓ cup (75 ml) white chocolate chips

1 egg, beaten

¼ cup (50 ml) unsalted peanuts

Makes 25 cookies

1 Preheat the oven to 375°F (190°C).

2 In a bowl, mix together the flour and the baking powder. Cut in the margarine with a knife, and work it with your fingertips until the mixture resembles fine bread crumbs.

3 Stir in the sugar, peanut butter and chocolate, and mix well.

4 Mix in the egg to make a firm dough (you will find it easier to use your hands as the mixture gets firmer).

5 Form the dough into 25 equal-size balls and press them onto a lightly floured cookie sheet. Press down each one with the back of a fork to make a pattern.

6 Decorate the top with the peanuts and bake for 10–12 minutes until golden brown. Cool on a wire rack.

FRUIT & NUT COOKIES
For a lower-fat alternative, you could use chopped apricots or dark raisins as a substitute for the white chocolate.

LOW-SUGAR SHORTBREAD

Though it is considerably lower in sugar and fat than most shortbreads, this still has a delicious buttery flavor. The rice flour gives it a satisfyingly crunchy texture.

1 Preheat the oven to 300°F (150°C).

2 Lightly grease an 8-inch (20-cm) round pan and line it with parchment paper.

3 Cream the butter until it is light and fluffy, then beat in the sugar.

4 Add the sifted flour and rice flour, a little at a time, and mix lightly each time. Shape the dough into a circle to fit the prepared pan.

5 Crimp the edges with the handle of a fork, cut into 8 wedges and bake in the center of the oven until golden, about 35–40 minutes.

6 Remove the lining paper, dust with sugar and cool on a wire rack.

⅓ cup (75 ml) butter

3 tablespoons (45 ml) granulated sugar

¾ cup (175 ml) all-purpose flour

½ cup (125 ml) rice flour

1 tablespoon (15 ml) granulated sugar, to decorate

Makes 8 pieces

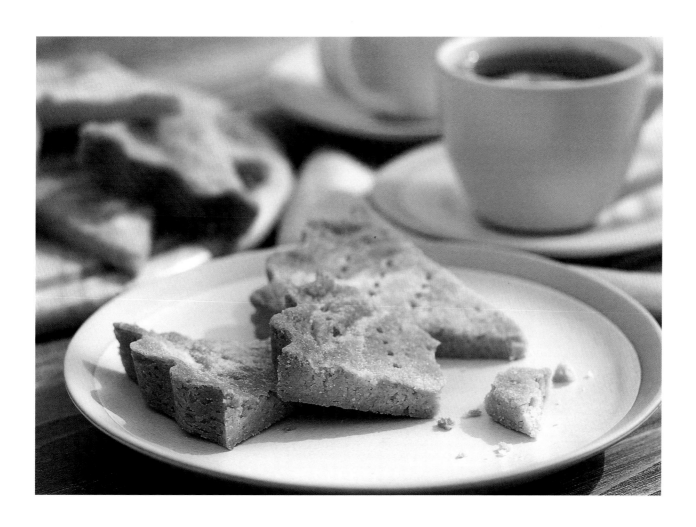

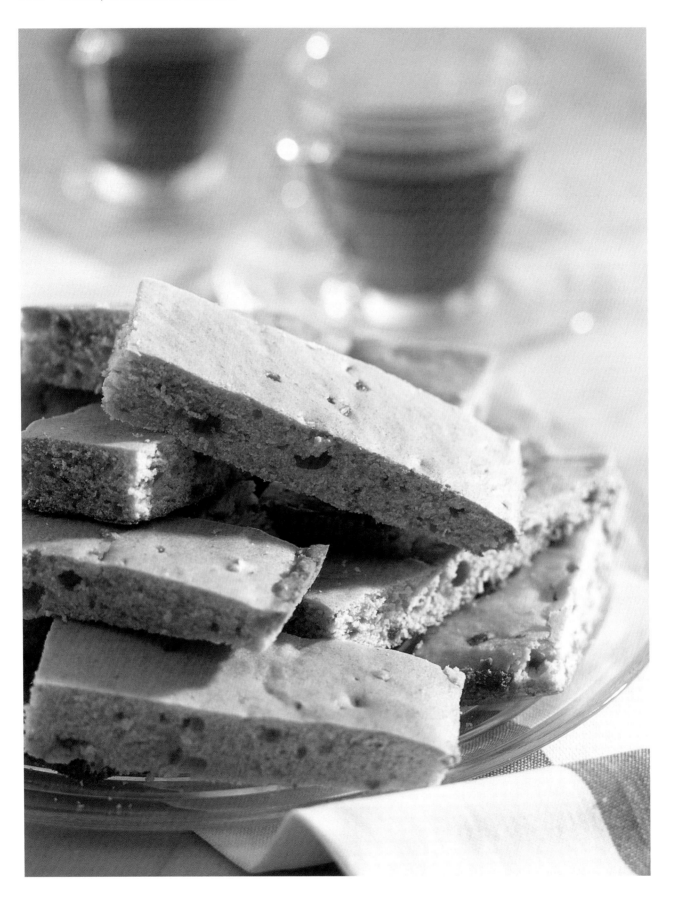

CHERRY ALMOND BARS

You'll certainly enjoy the aromas of almonds and cherries while these delicious homemade bars are baking in the oven. They're easy to cook and even easier to eat, making this a perfect afternoon treat.

1 Preheat the oven to 325°F (170°C). Lightly grease and line a jelly-roll pan with parchment paper.

2 Sift the flour and baking powder. In a large bowl, cream the margarine and sugar until light and fluffy. Stir in the ground almonds and cherries.

3 Mix the beaten egg with the milk and almond extract, and gradually beat into the creamed margarine and sugar, adding a little of the flour mixture if there is any sign of curdling.

4 Beat in the rest of the flour mixture, turn into the prepared pan and bake for about 35 minutes or until a skewer inserted in the center comes out clean.

5 Remove the lining paper, allow to cool on a wire rack and when completely cool, cut into bars or squares before serving.

2 cups (500 ml) all-purpose flour

2 teaspoons (10 ml) baking powder

⅔ cup (150 ml) reduced-fat margarine

2 tablespoons (25 ml) granulated sugar

⅔ cup (175 ml) ground almonds

⅓ cup, plus 2 tbsp (100 ml) candied cherries, finely chopped

1 large egg, beaten

¾ cup (175 ml) skim milk

1 teaspoon (5 ml) almond extract

Makes 16 bars

FRUITY FLAPJACK SQUARES

These flapjack squares are crammed with fruit and make great snacks, as they also contain oats to stabilize your blood glucose. Any mixture of fruit can be used—try prunes or raisins, or add some sesame or sunflower seeds for a different flavor and texture.

1 Preheat the oven to 350°F (180°C).

2 Mix the rolled oats, dried fruit and cinnamon together in a large bowl.

3 Place the butter and sugar in a saucepan, and stir over a low heat until the sugar is melted.

4 Add to the oat mixture and stir thoroughly until it is well combined.

5 Press the mixture into a non-stick baking pan (about 7 inches (18 cm) square).

6 Bake for about 25 minutes until lightly browned.

7 Leave to cool in the pan and cut into squares when still slightly warm.

2 cups (500 ml) rolled oats

⅓ cup, plus 2 tablespoons (100 ml) dried apricots, chopped

⅓ cup (75 ml) dried pineapple, chopped

⅓ cup (75 ml) dried banana chips, chopped

½ cup (125 ml) dried mango, chopped

⅓ cup, plus 2 tablespoons (100 ml) dried cranberries

½ teaspoon (2 ml) ground cinnamon

½ cup (125 ml) butter

⅔ cup (150 ml) light brown sugar

Makes 25 flapjack squares

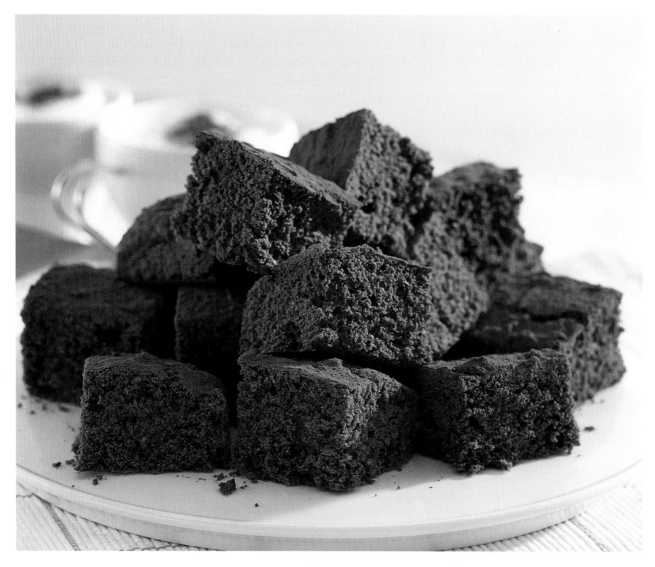

CHOCOLATE BROWNIES

These moist, chocolate-flavored treats are perfect just as they are, and they certainly don't need the traditional coating of sugary icing.

1 cup (250 ml) all-purpose flour	

1 cup (250 ml) all-purpose flour

1 cup (250 ml) wholewheat flour

Pinch of salt

2½ teaspoons (12 ml) baking powder

½ cup (100 ml) cocoa powder, plus additional for dusting

¾ cup (175 ml) reduced-fat margarine

¼ cup (50 ml) granulated sugar

2 medium eggs, beaten

⅓ cup, plus 2 tablespoons (100 ml) skim milk

Makes 16 brownies

1 Preheat the oven to 350°F (180°C).

2 Lightly grease an 8-inch (20-cm) square cake pan and line the base with parchment paper.

3 Sift the flours, salt, baking powder and cocoa powder into a large bowl, tipping in any leftover bran in the sifter.

4 Cream the margarine and sugar together until light and fluffy.

5 Beat in the eggs, a little at a time, adding a little of the flour mixture if there is any sign of curdling. Add the rest of the flour and mix it in thoroughly. Add the milk and beat until smooth.

6 Spoon the batter into the prepared cake pan and bake for 25 minutes. Then, turn the oven down to 300°F (150°C), and bake for a further 15–20 minutes, or until a skewer inserted in the center comes out clean.

7 Cool in the pan for 15 minutes, peel off the lining paper and leave to cool completely on a wire rack.

8 Cut into 16 squares and dust with unsweetened cocoa powder before serving.

EASY IRISH SODA BREAD

This recipe is based on a traditional Irish soda bread. Because baking soda is used as the leavening agent, it will start to "work" very quickly when it mixes with the milk, so make sure that you have your oven heated and the baking sheet(s) greased before you start.

3 cups (750 ml) wholewheat flour
1 cup (250 ml) unbleached all-purpose flour
½ teaspoon (2 ml) salt
1 teaspoon (5 ml) baking soda
4 teaspoons (20 ml) margarine
1¼ cups (300 ml) buttermilk
Serves 12 (makes 2 loaves, each serving 6)

1 Preheat the oven to 450°F (230°C) and lightly grease 1 large (or 2 medium-sized) baking sheets.

2 Sift both the flours with the salt and baking soda into a large bowl. Set aside any bran remaining in the sifter.

3 Lightly rub in the margarine, add the buttermilk and mix quickly to a soft but manageable dough. If it's too dry to handle, add a little water.

4 Turn-out onto a lightly floured board and knead for 1 minute or so, then cut in half and shape into 2 rounds.

5 Roll out the rounds to about 1 inch (2½ cm) thickness, and place them onto the greased baking sheet(s).

6 Score each round quite deeply to make 6 wedges in each. Sprinkle lightly with the reserved bran and bake the loaves for about 25 minutes, or until risen and golden.

7 Cool on a wire rack.

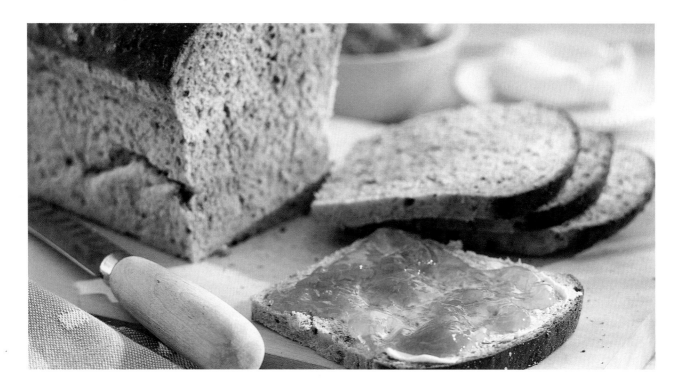

Farmhouse Whole-grain Bread

It's very satisfying to make your own bread, and this whole-grain loaf has a wonderfully evocative aroma while it's baking. A small egg white is used to glaze the top, but this is optional—it does, however, give a more attractive glossy appearance. Serve the bread warm or cold, but for best results bring it to the table when it's still warm, and watch how quickly it disappears.

4⅓ cups (1050 ml) stoneground wholewheat flour

Pinch of salt

1½ teaspoons (7 g) dry yeast

2 tablespoons (25 ml) sunflower oil

1¼ cups (300 ml) warm water

1 small egg white, lightly beaten (optional)

Makes a 2 lb (900 g) loaf (15 slices)

1   Put the flour and salt into a large bowl, then add the yeast and mix well.

2   Add the oil and water and mix thoroughly to make a pliable dough (if it is too dry to handle easily, add a little extra water).

3   Knead the dough for about 6–8 minutes, or until it is smooth and elastic.

4   Shape the dough to fit an 8 x 4 inch (1.5 liter) lightly greased loaf pan, lined with parchment paper. Cover it with a clean dish towel and leave in a warm place for about 1 hour or until it has doubled in size.

5   Preheat the oven to 450°F (230°C).

6   Brush the top of the bread with the lightly beaten egg white and bake for 30–35 minutes until it is golden.

7   Turn out of pan and cool on a wire rack. Serve with margarine and reduced-sugar jam, if desired.

Nutritional Analysis

The nutritional information for each recipe refers to a single serving, unless otherwise stated. Optional ingredients are not included. The figures are intended as a guide only. If salt is given in a measured amount in the recipe it has been included in the analysis; if the recipe suggests adding a pinch of salt or seasoning to taste, salt has not been included.

Recipe Name	Nutrient Information				Canadian Diabetes Association Food Choice Value		American Diabetes Association Exchanges	
p. 12 Oatmeal Cookies with Raisins & Sour Cherries 1 cookie/ 1/25 of recipe	102	Calories	15 g	Carbohydrate	1	Starch	1	Starch
	2 g	Protein	1 g	Fiber	1	Fats & Oils	1	Fat
	4 g	Fat	19 mg	Cholesterol				
	3 g	Saturated fat	115 mg	Sodium				
p. 12 Homemade Crunchy Muesli 1/14 of recipe	192	Calories	30 g	Carbohydrate	1	Starch	1	Starch
	5 g	Protein	4 g	Fiber	1	Fruits & Vegetables	2/3	Fruit
	7 g	Fat	0 mg	Cholesterol	1/2	Protein	1	Fat
	1 g	Saturated fat	5 mg	Sodium	1	Fats & Oils		
p. 13 Apricot Bran Breakfast Muffins 1 muffin/ 1/8 of recipe	176	Calories	28 g	Carbohydrate	1	Starch	1	Starch
	4 g	Protein	5 g	Fiber	1/2	Fruits & Vegetables	1/2	Fruit
	7 g	Fat	27 mg	Cholesterol			1/2	Other Carbohydrate
	1 g	Saturated fat	130 mg	Sodium	1/2	Sugars		
					1 1/2	Fats & Oils	1 1/2	Fat
p. 14 Fruity Breakfast Pancakes 1 pancake/ 1/8 of recipe	135	Calories	16 g	Carbohydrate	1	Starch	1	Starch
	3 g	Protein	1 g	Fiber	1 1/2	Fats & Oils	1 1/2	Fat
	7 g	Fat	27 mg	Cholesterol				
	1 g	Saturated fat	178 mg	Sodium				
p. 15 Honey-grilled Grapefruit with Toasted Sesame Seeds 1/4 of recipe	71	Calories	13 g	Carbohydrate	1	Fruits & Vegetables	1/2	Fruit
	1 g	Protein	0 g	Fiber			1/2	Other Carbohydrate
	2 g	Fat	0 mg	Cholesterol	1/2	Sugars		
	0 g	Saturated fat	2 mg	Sodium	1/2	Fats & Oils	1/2	Fat
p. 15 Banana & Mango Yogurt Smoothie with Wheatgerm 1/2 of recipe	293	Calories	59 g	Carbohydrate	3	Fruits & Vegetables	2	Fruit
	12 g	Protein	5 g	Fiber			1	Low Fat Milk
	4 g	Fat	7 mg	Cholesterol	2	1% Milk	2/3	Other Carbohydrate
	2 g	Saturated fat	115 mg	Sodium	1	Sugars		
					1/2	Fats & Oils		

Recipe Name	Nutrient Information			Canadian Diabetes Association Food Choice Value		American Diabetes Association Exchanges	
p. 16 Scrambled Eggs with Smoked Salmon $1/4$ of recipe	132 Calories 12 g Protein 8 g Fat 2 g Saturated fat	4 g 1 g 222 mg 390 mg	Carbohydrate Fiber Cholesterol Sodium	$1/2$ $1^1/2$ $1/2$	Fruits & Vegetables Protein Fats & Oils	$1/2$ $1^1/2$	Vegetable Medium-Fat Meat
p. 16 Eggs Florentine $1/4$ of recipe	228 Calories 13 g Protein 11 g Fat 5 g Saturated fat	20 g 2 g 229 mg 323 m	Carbohydrate Fiber Cholesterol Sodium	1 $1^1/2$ $1^1/2$ 1	Starch Protein Fats & Oils Extras	1 $1/2$ $1^1/2$ 1	Starch Vegetable Medium-Fat Meat Fat
p. 17 Salmon Kedgeree with Fresh Cilantro $1/4$ of recipe	414 Calories 25 g Protein 12 g Fat 2 g Saturated fat	43 g 1 g 156 mg 73 mg	Carbohydrate Fiber Cholesterol Sodium	3 $2^1/2$ 2	Starch Protein Fats & Oils (one from EtOH)	3 2 1	Starch Lean Meat Fat
p. 19 Smoked Haddock Soufflé Omelet with Croutons $1/2$ of recipe	415 Calories 35 g Protein 23 g Fat 7 g Saturated fat	17 g 2 g 407 mg 958 mg	Carbohydrate Fiber Cholesterol Sodium	1 $4^1/2$ 2	Starch Protein Fats & Oils	1 $4^1/2$ 2	Starch Lean Meat Fat
p. 20 Wild Mushroom Toasts $1/4$ of recipe	323 Calories 10 g Protein 10 g Fat 2 g Saturated fat	54 g 5 g 3 mg 164 mg	Carbohydrate Fiber Cholesterol Sodium	2 2 $1/2$ 2	Starch Fruits & Vegetables Protein Fats & Oils	2 4 2	Starch Vegetable Fat
p. 21 Potato Cakes $1/12$ of recipe	50 Calories 1 g Protein 0 g Fat 0 g Saturated fat	10 g 1 g 0 mg 38 mg	Carbohydrate Fiber Cholesterol Sodium	$1/2$	Starch	$1/2$	Starch
p. 24 Shrimp & Apple Pita Pockets $1/4$ of recipe	198 Calories 15 g Protein 3 g Fat 0 g Saturated fat	28 g 1 g 61 mg 759 mg	Carbohydrate Fiber Cholesterol Sodium	1 1 $1^1/2$ 1	Starch Fruits & Vegetables Protein Extras	1 1 2	Starch Fruit Very Lean Meat
p. 24 Layered Mediterranean Sandwich $1/4$ of recipe	247 Calories 11 g Protein 9 g Fat 4 g Saturated fat	32 g 3 g 24 mg 468 mg	Carbohydrate Fiber Cholesterol Sodium	$1^1/2$ $1/2$ 1 1	Starch Fruits & Vegetables Protein Fats & Oils	$1^1/2$ 1 1 $1/2$	Starch Vegetable Medium-Fat Meat Fat

Recipe Name	Nutrient Information				Canadian Diabetes Association Food Choice Value		American Diabetes Association Exchanges	
p. 25 Goat Cheese, Tomato & Ciabatta Grill $^1/_2$ of recipe	595 28 g 29 g 16 g	Calories Protein Fat Saturated fat	56 g 4 g 62 mg 819 mg	Carbohydrate Fiber Cholesterol Sodium	$3^1/_2$ 3 4	Starch Protein Fats & Oils	$3^1/_2$ $2^1/_2$ $1^1/_2$	Starch Lean Meat Fat
p. 26 Portuguese Sardine Salad $^1/_6$ of recipe	553 45 g 25 g 3 g	Calories Protein Fat Saturated fat	37 g 5 g 237 mg 983 mg	Carbohydrate Fiber Cholesterol Sodium	2 $5^1/_2$ 2 1	Starch Protein Fats & Oils Extras	2 $5^1/_2$ 2	Starch Lean Meat Fat
p. 26 Tuna & Dill Dip with Vegetable Crudités $^1/_4$ of recipe	157 16 g 3 g 1 g	Calories Protein Fat Saturated fat	18 g 4 g 24 mg 315 mg	Carbohydrate Fiber Cholesterol Sodium	$1^1/_2$ 2	Fruits & Vegetables Protein	3 $1^1/_2$	Vegetable Lean Meat
p. 27 Avocado with Chicken & Walnut Salad $^1/_4$ of recipe	602 31 g 47 g 7 g	Calories Protein Fat Saturated fat	20 g 6 g 65 mg 58 mg	Carbohydrate Fiber Cholesterol Sodium	$1^1/_2$ 4 7	Fruits & Vegetables Protein Fats & Oils	1 $4^1/_2$ $8^1/_2$	Fruit Very Lean Meat Fat
p. 28 Warm Lentils & Kidney Beans with Bacon $^1/_4$ of recipe	414 28 g 13 g 3 g	Calories Protein Fat Saturated fat	48 g 10 g 22 mg 566 mg	Carbohydrate Fiber Cholesterol Sodium	$2^1/_2$ $3^1/_2$ $^1/_2$	Starch Protein Fats & Oils	$2^1/_2$ 3 1	Starch Lean Meet Fat
p. 28 Sweet Potato & Vegetable Stew $^1/_4$ of recipe	303 13 g 5 g 1 g	Calories Protein Fat Saturated fat	56 g 11 g 0 m 26 mg	Carbohydrate Fiber Cholesterol Sodium	2 $1^1/_2$ 1 $^1/_2$	Starch Fruits & Vegetables Protein Fats & Oils	2 3 $^1/_2$ 1	Starch Vegetable Very Low Fat Meat Fat
p. 29 Tuscan Bread Salad with Red Onion & Mozzarella $^1/_4$ of recipe	400 18 g 20 g 7 g	Calories Protein Fat Saturated fat	39 g 4 g 24 mg 562 mg	Carbohydrate Fiber Cholesterol Sodium	$1^1/_2$ 1 2 $2^1/_2$ 1	Starch Fruits & Vegetables Protein Fats & Oils Extras	$1^1/_2$ 2 2 2	Starch Vegetable Medium-Fat Meat Fat
p. 29 Homemade Popcorn $^1/_4$ of recipe	56 1 g 2 g 0 g	Calories Protein Fat Saturated fat	9 g 2 g 0 mg 0 mg	Carbohydrate Fiber Cholesterol Sodium	$^1/_2$ $^1/_2$	Starch Fats & Oils	$^1/_2$ $^1/_2$	Starch Fat

Recipe Name	Nutrient Information			Canadian Diabetes Association Food Choice Value		American Diabetes Association Exchanges	
p. 31 Potato, Red Pepper & Onion Frittata ¹/₄ of recipe	158 Calories 8 g Protein 9 g Fat 2 g Saturated fat	13 g 2 g 216 mg 64 mg	Carbohydrate Fiber Cholesterol Sodium	¹/₂ ¹/₂ 1 1	Starch Fruits & Vegetables Protein Fats & Oils	¹/₂ 1 ¹/₂ ¹/₂	Starch Vegetable Medium-Fat Meat Fat
p. 31 Vegetable Gratin ¹/₄ of recipe	137 Calories 7 g Protein 4 g Fat 2 g Saturated fat	20 g 5 g 8 mg 491 mg	Carbohydrate Fiber Cholesterol Sodium	1¹/₂ 1	Fruits & Vegetables Protein	3 1	Vegetable Fat
p. 32 Pizza with Tri-colored Peppers & Beans ¹/₄ of recipe	484 Calories 23 g Protein 12 g Fat 4 g Saturated fat	75 g 8 g 16 mg 820 mg	Carbohydrate Fiber Cholesterol Sodium	2¹/₂ 3 2 1	Starch Fruits & Vegetables Protein Fats & Oils	2¹/₂ 5 ¹/₂ 2	Starch Vegetable Medium-Fat Meat Fat
p. 34 Stuffed Baked Potatoes ¹/₄ of recipe	303 Calories 6 g Protein 4 g Fat 0 g Saturated fat	63 g 6 g 0 mg 19 mg	Carbohydrate Fiber Cholesterol Sodium	4 1	Starch Fats & Oils	4 1	Starch Fat
p. 34 Stuffed Baked Potatoes: Avocado with Shrimp ¹/₄ of recipe	417 Calories 12 g Protein 12 g Fat 2 g Saturated fat	68 g 7 g 38 mg 74 mg	Carbohydrate Fiber Cholesterol Sodium	4 ¹/₂ 2	Starch Protein Fats & Oils	4 2¹/₂	Starch Fat
p. 34 Stuffed Baked Potatoes: Tuna Tricolor ¹/₄ of recipe	378 Calories 13 g Protein 7 g Fat 1 g Saturated fat	68 g 6 g 12 mg 125 mg	Carbohydrate Fiber Cholesterol Sodium	4 1 ¹/₂ 1	Starch Protein Fats & Oils Extra	4 1¹/₂	Starch Fat
p. 34 Stuffed Baked Potatoes: Smoked Ham with Pesto Sauce ¹/₄ of recipe	502 Calories 16 g Protein 21 g Fat 5 g Saturated fat	66 g 6 g 20 mg 542 mg	Carbohydrate Fiber Cholesterol Sodium	4 1 3 ¹/₂	Starch Protein Fats & Oils	4 ¹/₂ 4	Starch Lean Meat Fat
p. 35 Baked Cheesy Triangles ¹/₄ of recipe	235 Calories 15 g Protein 7 g Fat 4 g Saturated fat	29 g 4 g 16 mg 441 mg	Carbohydrate Fiber Cholesterol Sodium	1¹/₂ ¹/₂ 1¹/₂ ¹/₂	Starch 2% Milk Protein Fats & Oils	1¹/₂ 1¹/₂ ¹/₂	Starch Medium-Fat Meat Fat

Recipe Name	Nutrient Information				Canadian Diabetes Association Food Choice Value		American Diabetes Association Exchanges	
p. 35 Stuffed Peppers ¹/₄ of recipe	246 8 g 4 g 1 g	Calories Protein Fat Saturated fat	46 g 5 g 4 mg 75 mg	Carbohydrate Fiber Cholesterol Sodium	2 1 ¹/₂ ¹/₂	Starch Fruits & Vegetables Protein Fats & Oils	2 2 1	Starch Vegetable Fat
p. 38 Pumpkin Soup with Roast Parsnip Chips ¹/₄ of recipe	207 5 g 7 g 1 g	Calories Protein Fat Saturated fat	36 g 5 g 0 mg 628 mg	Carbohydrate Fiber Cholesterol Sodium	3 1¹/₂	Fruits & Vegetables Fats & Oils	6 1¹/₂	Vegetable Fat
p. 39 Bean & Pasta Soup with Basil ¹/₄ of recipe	278 14 g 12 g 2 g	Calories Protein Fat Saturated fat	30 g 3 g 2 mg 1102 mg	Carbohydrate Fiber Cholesterol Sodium	1 1 1¹/₂ 1¹/₂ 1	Starch Fruits & Vegetables Protein Fats & Oils Extras	1 2 1 2	Starch Vegetable Very Lean Meat Fat
p. 40 Red Lentil Soup ¹/₄ of recipe	255 20 g 1 g 0 g	Calories Protein Fat Saturated fat	43 g 9 g 7 mg 99 mg	Carbohydrate Fiber Cholesterol Sodium	1¹/₂ 1 2¹/₂	Starch Fruits & Vegetables Protein	1¹/₂ 2 2	Starch Vegetable Very Low Fat Meat
p. 40 Spinach & Onion Soup ¹/₄ of recipe	141 6 g 6 g 1 g	Calories Protein Fat Saturated fat	14 g 3 g 0 mg 1011 mg	Carbohydrate Fiber Cholesterol Sodium	1 1 ¹/₂	Fruits & Vegetables Protein Fats & Oils	2 1	Vegetable Fat
p. 41 Fish & Potato Soup ¹/₄ of recipe	294 35 g 3 g 2 g	Calories Protein Fat Saturated fat	30 g 3 g 95 mg 988 mg	Carbohydrate Fiber Cholesterol Sodium	1¹/₂ ¹/₂ 4¹/₂	Starch Fruits & Vegetables Protein	1¹/₂ 1 4	Starch Vegetable Very Lean Meat
p. 41 Garlic Bread ¹/₄ of recipe	186 5 g 7 g 1 g	Calories Protein Fat Saturated fat	26 g 1 g 0 mg 415 mg	Carbohydrate Fiber Cholesterol Sodium	1¹/₂ 1¹/₂	Starch Fats & Oils	1¹/₂ 1¹/₂	Starch Fat
p. 43 Garlic Tiger Shrimp ¹/₄ of recipe	92 12 g 4 g 1 g	Calories Protein Fat Saturated fat	1 g 0 g 86 mg 80 mg	Carbohydrate Fiber Cholesterol Sodium	1¹/₂	Protein	1¹/₂ ¹/₂	Very Lean Meat Fat
p. 43 Monkfish Kabobs with Lemon & Thyme ¹/₄ of recipe	172 24 g 6 g 1 g	Calories Protein Fat Saturated fat	6 g 1 g 41 mg 30 mg	Carbohydrate Fiber Cholesterol Sodium	¹/₂ 3¹/₂	Fruits & Vegetables Protein	1 3¹/₂ ¹/₂	Vegetable Very Lean Meat Fat

Recipe Name	Nutrient Information			Canadian Diabetes Association Food Choice Value		American Diabetes Association Exchanges	
p. 44 Honey-glazed Chicken Wings 1/4 of recipe	346 Calories 27 g Protein 24 g Fat 7 g Saturated fat	5 g 0 g 113 mg 138 mg	Carbohydrate Fiber Cholesterol Sodium	1/2 4 2 1/2	Sugar Protein Fats & Oils	1/3 4 1/2	Other Carbohydrate Medium-Fat Meat Fat
p. 44 Sautéed Chicken Liver with Fennel 1/4 of recipe	112 Calories 11 g Protein 5 g Fat 1 g Saturated fat	7 g 0 g 247 mg 73 mg	Carbohydrate Fiber Cholesterol Sodium	1/2 1 1/2	Fruits & Vegetables Protein	1 1	Vegetable Lean Meat
p. 45 Mini Kabobs with Yogurt Dip 1/4 of recipe	243 Calories 15 g Protein 18 g Fat 0 g Saturated fat	4 g 0 g 57 mg 344 mg	Carbohydrate Fiber Cholesterol Sodium	1/2 2 2	2% Milk Protein Fats & Oils	1/4 2 1 1/2	Low Fat Milk Medium-Fat Meat Fat
p. 46 Falafels with Mint Dip 12 falafels (1 falafel)	62 Calories 3 g Protein 1 g Fat 0 g Saturated fat	10 g 0 g 1 mg 187 mg	Carbohydrate Fiber Cholesterol Sodium	1/2 1/2	Starch Fruits & Vegetables	2/3	Starch
p. 46 Roasted Baby Tomatoes & Eggplant 1/4 of recipe	56 Calories 2 g Protein 1 g Fat 0 g Saturated fat	13 g 2 g 0 mg 14 mg	Carbohydrate Fiber Cholesterol Sodium	1	Fruits & Vegetables	2	Vegetable
p. 47 Crispy Potato Wedges with Cream & Chive Dip 1/4 of recipe	189 Calories 5 g Protein 9 g Fat 1 g Saturated fat	23 g 2 g 4 mg 36 mg	Carbohydrate Fiber Cholesterol Sodium	1 1 1	Starch Whole Milk Fats & Oils	1 1/2 1	Starch Whole Milk Fat
p. 50 Tiger Shrimp Risotto 1/4 of recipe	493 Calories 33 g Protein 7 g Fat 3 g Saturated fat	73 g 4 g 160 mg 1683 mg	Carbohydrate Fiber Cholesterol Sodium	3 2 1/2 3 1/2	Starch Fruits & Vegetables Protein	3 5 2 1	Starch Vegetable Protein Fat
p. 51 Stir-fried Squid with Lemon Grass & Ginger 1/4 of recipe	379 Calories 28 g Protein 8 g Fat 1 g Saturated fat	50 g 4 g 316 mg 272 mg	Carbohydrate Fiber Cholesterol Sodium	2 1/2 1 3	Starch Fruits & Vegetables Protein	2 1/2 2 2 1/2 1	Starch Vegetable Very Low Fat Meat Fat

Recipe Name	Nutrient Information			Canadian Diabetes Association Food Choice Value		American Diabetes Association Exchanges	
p. 51 Smoked Fish Parcels $^1/_4$ of recipe	190 Calories 30 g Protein 2 g Fat 0 g Saturated fat	10 g 1 g 0 mg 1207 mg	Carbohydrate Fiber Cholesterol Sodium	$^1/_2$ 4	Starch Protein	$^1/_2$ 4	Starch Very Lean Meat
p. 52 Pan-Fried Cod with Pesto $^1/_4$ of recipe	502 Calories 42 g Protein 36 g Fat 6 g Saturated fat	6 g 0 g 92 mg 250 mg	Carbohydrate Fiber Cholesterol Sodium	$^1/_2$ 6 $3^1/_2$	Fruits & Vegetables Protein Fats & Oils	1 6 6	Vegetable Very Lean Meat Fat
p. 52 Balsamic Salmon Steaks $^1/_4$ of recipe	290 Calories 36 g Protein 15 g Fat 2 g Saturated fat	2 g 0 g 96 mg 595 mg	Carbohydrate Fiber Cholesterol Sodium	7 1	Protein Extra	7	Lean Meat
p. 53 Grilled Halibut Steaks with Red Pepper Sauce $^1/_4$ of recipe	262 Calories 37 g Protein 10 g Fat 1 g Saturated fat	4 g 1 g 56 mg 139 mg	Carbohydrate Fiber Cholesterol Sodium	$^1/_2$ 7	Fruits & Vegetables Protein	1 7 $^1/_2$	Vegetable Very Low Fat Meat Fat
p. 54 Fettuccine with Salmon, Asparagus & Lemon $^1/_4$ of recipe	590 Calories 40 g Protein 14 g Fat 3 g Saturated fat	75 g 3 g 74 mg 100 mg	Carbohydrate Fiber Cholesterol Sodium	4 1 $4^1/_2$	Starch Fruits & Vegetables Protein	4 2 4 $^1/_2$	Starch Vegetable Low Fat Meat Fat
p. 56 Coriander Chicken with Orange $^1/_4$ of recipe	297 Calories 18 g Protein 15 g Fat 2 g Saturated fat	26 g 4 g 52 mg 238 mg	Carbohydrate Fiber Cholesterol Sodium	2 $2^1/_2$ $1^1/_2$ 1	Fruits & Vegetables Protein Fats & Oils Extra	1 1 $2^1/_2$ $1^1/_2$	Fruit Vegetable Lean Meat Fat
p. 56 Chicken Breasts with Salsa $^1/_2$ of recipe	454 Calories 39 g Protein 26 g Fat 4 g Saturated fat	22 g 5 g 87 mg 127 mg	Carbohydrate Fiber Cholesterol Sodium	$1^1/_2$ $5^1/_2$ 2 1	Fruits & Vegetables Protein Fats & Oils Extras	3 $4^1/_2$ 4	Vegetable Very Low Fat Low Meat Fat
p. 57 Chicken with Ginger $^1/_4$ of recipe	297 Calories 40 g Protein 6 g Fat 1 g Saturated fat	19 g 0 g 102 mg 494 mg	Carbohydrate Fiber Cholesterol Sodium	$^1/_2$ 1 $5^1/_2$	Starch Sugar Protein	$^1/_2$ $^2/_3$ $5^1/_2$	Starch Other Carbohydrate Very Lean Meat

Recipe Name	Nutrient Information				Canadian Diabetes Association Food Choice Value		American Diabetes Association Exchanges	
p. 58 Chicken with Cardamom ¹/₄ of recipe	346 Calories 27 g Protein 13 g Fat 2 g Saturated fat	34 g Carbohydrate 5 g Fiber 47 mg Cholesterol 251 mg Sodium			¹/₂ Starch 1¹/₂ Fruits & Vegetables 1 2% Milk 3 Protein ¹/₂ Fats & Oils		¹/₂ Starch 1 Fruit ¹/₂ Low Fat Milk 3 Very Low Fat Meat 1¹/₂ Fat	
p. 58 Turkey with Red Onion & Watercress Salad ¹/₄ of recipe	316 Calories 44 g Protein 8 g Fat 1 g Saturated fat	16 g Carbohydrate 3 g Fiber 105 mg Cholesterol 94 mg Sodium			1¹/₂ Fruits & Vegetables 6 Protein		²/₃ Fruit 1 Vegetable 6 Very Low Fat Meat ¹/₂ Fat	
p. 60 Turkey Fricassee with Olive Oil Mashed Potatoes ¹/₄ of recipe	502 Calories 49 g Protein 17 g Fat 3 g Saturated fat	38 g Carbohydrate 4 g Fiber 111 mg Cholesterol 767 mg Sodium			1¹/₂ Starch 1 Fruits & Vegetables 6¹/₂ Protein		1¹/₂ Starch 2 Vegetable 6 Very Low Fat Meat 2 Fat	
p. 61 Duck Breasts with Coconut ¹/₄ of recipe	304 Calories 18 g Protein 22 g Fat 17 g Saturated fat	11 g Carbohydrate 2 g Fiber 58 mg Cholesterol 154 mg Sodium			1 Fruits & Vegetables 2¹/₂ Protein 3 Fats & Oils		2 Vegetable 2 Low Fat Meat 3 Fat	
p. 61 Sweet & Sour Duck ¹/₄ of recipe	300 Calories 24 g Protein 8 g Fat 2 g Saturated fat	31 g Carbohydrate 3 g Fiber 89 mg Cholesterol 810 mg Sodium			2¹/₂ Fruits & Vegetables ¹/₂ Sugars 3 Protein		1 Fruit 3 Vegetable 3 Low Fat Meat	
p. 62 Smoked Sausage Cassoulet ¹/₄ of recipe	465 Calories 30 g Protein 11 g Fat 4 g Saturated fat	64 g Carbohydrate 13 g Fiber 44 mg Cholesterol 2035 mg Sodium			1¹/₂ Starch 3 Fruits & Vegetables 3¹/₂ Protein		1¹/₂ Starch 6 Vegetable 2 High Fat Meat	
p. 62 Italian Meatballs ¹/₄ of recipe	690 Calories 32 g Protein 24 g Fat 8 g Saturated fat	83 g Carbohydrate 6 g Fiber 72 mg Cholesterol 166 mg Sodium			4¹/₂ Starch 1 Fruits & Vegetables 3 Protein 3 Fats & Oils		4¹/₂ Starch 2 Vegetable 2 High Fat Meat 1¹/₂ Fat	
p. 64 Beef with Green Pepper & Noodles ¹/₄ of recipe	621 Calories 40 g Protein 16 g Fat 3 g Saturated fat	78 g Carbohydrate 5 g Fiber 60 mg Cholesterol 824 mg Sodium			4 Starch 1¹/₂ Fruits & Vegetables 4 Protein ¹/₂ Fats & Oils		4 Starch 3 Vegetable 3 Lean Meat 1¹/₂ Fat	

Recipe Name	Nutrient Information			Canadian Diabetes Association Food Choice Value		American Diabetes Association Exchanges	
p. 64 Grilled Beef Tenderloin with Wild Mushrooms ¹/₄ of recipe	302 Calories 28 g Protein 16 g Fat 8 g Saturated fat	12 g 2 g 62 mg 120 mg	Carbohydrate Fiber Cholesterol Sodium	1 4 1	Fruits & Vegetables Protein Fats & Oils	2 3¹/₂ 1	Vegetable Lean Meat Fat
p. 65 Lamb with Apricots ¹/₄ of recipe	330 Calories 24 g Protein 7 g Fat 2 g Saturated fat	47 g 4 g 66 mg 463 mg	Carbohydrate Fiber Cholesterol Sodium	4¹/₂ 3	Fruits & Vegetables Protein	1¹/₂ 4 2¹/₂	Fruit Vegetable Lean Meat
p. 66 Lamb Baked in Yogurt ¹/₆ of recipe	652 Calories 85 g Protein 26 g Fat 8 g Saturated fat	17 g 2 g 250 mg 660 mg	Carbohydrate Fiber Cholesterol Sodium	1 1 11¹/₂	Fruits & Vegetables 2% Milk Protein	2 ¹/₂ 11	Vegetable Low Fat Milk Lean Meat
p. 66 Venison in Red Wine ¹/₄ of recipe	282 Calories 36 g Protein 9 g Fat 2 g Saturated fat	8 g 2 g 128 mg 316 mg	Carbohydrate Fiber Cholesterol Sodium	¹/₂ 5 1	Fruits & Vegetables Protein Extras	1 5 1	Vegetable Very Low Fat Meat Fat
p. 67 Broccoli & Herb Pasta ¹/₄ of recipe	405 Calories 17 g Protein 7 g Fat 2 g Saturated fat	71 g 6 g 5 mg 387 mg	Carbohydrate Fiber Cholesterol Sodium	3¹/₂ 1 1¹/₂ ¹/₂ 1	Starch Fruits & Vegetables Protein Fats & Oils Extras	3¹/₂ 2 ¹/₂ 1	Starch Vegetable Lean Meat Fat
p. 67 Vegetable Pilaf ¹/₄ of recipe	343 Calories 11 g Protein 3 g Fat 1 g Saturated fat	72 g 7 g 0 mg 369 mg	Carbohydrate Fiber Cholesterol Sodium	3 2 ¹/₂	Starch Fruits & Vegetables Fats & Oils	3 4 ¹/₂	Starch Vegetable Fat
p. 68 Polenta with Tomatoes, Porcini & Goat Cheese ¹/₂ of recipe	551 Calories 24 g Protein 28 g Fat 15 g Saturated fat	55 g 3 g 60 mg 1008 mg	Carbohydrate Fiber Cholesterol Sodium	2¹/₂ 1¹/₂ 2¹/₂ 4	Starch Fruits & Vegetables Protein Fats & Oils	2¹/₂ 4 1¹/₂ 4¹/₂	Starch Vegetable High Fat Meat Fat
p. 69 Polenta Bruschetta with Mediterranean Vegetables ¹/₄ of recipe	311 Calories 11 g Protein 10 g Fat 2 g Saturated fat	50 g 8 g 5 mg 366 mg	Carbohydrate Fiber Cholesterol Sodium	3 1¹/₂ 1 1	Starch Fruits & Vegetables Protein Extras	3 3 2	Starch Vegetable Fat

Recipe Name	Nutrient Information				Canadian Diabetes Association Food Choice Value		American Diabetes Association Exchanges	
p. 69 Mixed-pepper Couscous ¹/₄ of recipe	301 Calories 8 g Protein 7 g Fat 1 g Saturated fat	50 g Carbohydrate 3 g Fiber 0 mg Cholesterol 12 mg Sodium			2¹/₂ Starch 1 Fruits & Vegetables ¹/₂ Protein 1 Fats & Oils		2¹/₂ Starch 2 Vegetable 1¹/₂ Fat	
p. 70 Spicy Chickpeas in Wholewheat Wraps ¹/₄ of recipe	659 Calories 25 g Protein 16 g Fat 2 g Saturated fat	112 g Carbohydrate 19 g Fiber 1 mg Cholesterol 273 mg Sodium			6 Starch ¹/₂ Fruits & Vegetables 2 Protein 2 Fats & Oils		6 Starch 1 Vegetable ¹/₂ Very Low Fat Meat 3 Fat	
p. 72 Crepes Stuffed with Spinach & Ricotta ¹/₄ of recipe	296 Calories 20 g Protein 9 g Fat 4 g Saturated fat	37 g Carbohydrate 7 g Fiber 17 mg Cholesterol 346 mg Sodium			2 Starch 2 Protein ¹/₂ Fats & Oils		2 Starch 2 Low Fat Meat 1¹/₂ Fat	
p. 73 Penne with Roasted Vegetables ¹/₄ of recipe	394 Calories 11 g Protein 12 g Fat 2 g Saturated fat	63 g Carbohydrate 6 g Fiber 0 mg Cholesterol 19 mg Sodium			3 Starch 1 Fruits & Vegetables ¹/₂ Protein 2 Fats & Oils 1 Extras		3 Starch 2 Vegetable 2¹/₂ Fat	
p. 73 Saffron Rice with Vegetables & Soft Herb Cream Cheese ¹/₄ of recipe	372 Calories 10 g Protein 10 g Fat 4 Saturated fat	61 g Carbohydrate 3 g Fiber 19 mg Cholesterol 918 mg Sodium			3 Starch 1¹/₂ Fruits & Vegetables ¹/₂ Protein 1¹/₂ Fats & Oils		3 Starch 3 Vegetable 2 Fat	
p. 76 Lemon & Onion Roasted Potatoes ¹/₄ of recipe	199 Calories 4 g Protein 7 g Fat 1 g Saturated fat	34 g Carbohydrate 5 Fiber 0 mg Cholesterol 11 mg Sodium			2 Starch 1¹/₂ Fats & Oils		2 Starch 1¹/₂ Fat	
p. 76 Roasted New Potatoes with Tomatoes & Herbs ¹/₄ of recipe	131 Calories 3 g Protein 4 g Fat 1 g Saturated fat	23 g Carbohydrate 3 g Fiber 0 mg Cholesterol 14 mg Sodium			1 Starch ¹/₂ Fruits & Vegetables 1 Fats & Oils		1 Starch 1 Vegetable 1 Fat	
p. 78 Baked Sweet Potatoes with Spicy Butter ¹/₄ of recipe	229 Calories 4 g Protein 5 g Fat 3 g Saturated fat	61 g Carbohydrate 8 g Fiber 11 mg Cholesterol 77 mg Sodium			3¹/₂ Starch 1 Fats & Oils		3¹/₂ Starch 1 Fat	

Recipe Name	Nutrient Information				Canadian Diabetes Association Food Choice Value		American Diabetes Association Exchanges	
p. 78 Parsnip Croquettes $^1/_{20}$ of recipe (1 croquette)	45 1 g 0 g 0 g	Calories Protein Fat Saturated fat	9 g 1 g 11 mg 18 mg	Carbohydrate Fiber Cholesterol Sodium	$^1/_2$	Starch	$^1/_2$	Starch
p. 79 Corn Fritters $^1/_{15}$ of recipe (1 fritter)	51 2 g 1 g 0 g	Calories Protein Fat Saturated fat	10 g 1 g 14 mg 105 mg	Carbohydrate Fiber Cholesterol Sodium	$^1/_2$ 1	Starch Extra	$^1/_2$	Starch
p. 79 Stir-fried Baby Corn & Snow Peas $^1/_4$ of recipe	136 5 g 8 g 1 g	Calories Protein Fat Saturated fat	15 g 4 g 0 mg 11 mg	Carbohydrate Fiber Cholesterol Sodium	$^1/_2$ $^1/_2$ $^1/_2$ $1^1/_2$	Starch Fruits & Vegetables Protein Fats & Oils	$^1/_2$ 1 $1^1/_2$	Starch Vegetable Fat
p. 81 Roasted Mediterranean Vegetables with Pine Nuts $^1/_2$ of recipe	304 8 g 22 g 3 g	Calories Protein Fat Saturated fat	29 g 4 g 0 mg 28 mg	Carbohydrate Fiber Cholesterol Sodium	$2^1/_2$ 1 4	Fruits & Vegetables Protein Fats & Oils	5 $4^1/_2$	Vegetable Fat
p. 81 Baked Tomato & Olive Salad $^1/_4$ of recipe	60 1 g 5 g 1 g	Calories Protein Fat Saturated fat	4 g 1 g 0 mg 115 mg	Carbohydrate Fiber Cholesterol Sodium	$^1/_2$ 1	Fruits & Vegetables Fats & Oils	1 1	Vegetable Fat
p. 82 Tabouleh $^1/_4$ of recipe	203 6 g 8 g 1 g	Calories Protein Fat Saturated fat	32 g 5 g 0 mg 147 mg	Carbohydrate Fiber Cholesterol Sodium	1 1 $^1/_2$ 1 1	Starch Fruits & Vegetables Protein Fats & Oils Extra	1 2 $1^1/_2$	Starch Vegetable Fat
p. 83 Peppery Bean Salad $^1/_4$ of recipe	220 8 g 7 g 1 g	Calories Protein Fat Saturated fat	34 g 1 g 0 mg 436 mg	Carbohydrate Fiber Cholesterol Sodium	$1^1/_2$ 1 $^1/_2$ 1	Starch Fruits & Vegetables Protein Fats & Oils	$1^1/_2$ 2 $1^1/_2$	Starch Vegetable Fat
p. 83 Cabbage with Caraway Seeds $^1/_4$ of recipe	70 2 g 4 g 1 g	Calories Protein Fat Saturated fat	8 g 2 g 0 mg 20 mg	Carbohydrate Fiber Cholesterol Sodium	$^1/_2$ 1	Fruits & Vegetables Fats & Oils	1 1	Vegetable Fat

Recipe Name	Nutrient Information			Canadian Diabetes Association Food Choice Value		American Diabetes Association Exchanges	
p. 83 Red Cabbage Coleslaw ¹/₄ of recipe	125 Calories 2 g Protein 8 g Fat 0 g Saturated fat	14 g 3 g 0 mg 236 mg	Carbohydrate Fiber Cholesterol Sodium	1 1¹/₂	Fruits & Vegetables Fats & Oils	2 1¹/₂	Vegetable Fat
p. 86 Raspberry Soufflé Omelet ¹/₂ of recipe	201 Calories 6 g Protein 10 g Fat 2 g Saturated fat	23 g 1 g 216 mg 64 mg	Carbohydrate Fiber Cholesterol Sodium	2 1 1¹/₂	Sugars Protein Fats & Oils	1¹/₂ 1 1	Other Carbohydrate Medium Fat Meat Fat
p. 86 Baked Bananas with Orange ¹/₄ of recipe	137 Calories 1 g Protein 1 g Fat 0 g Saturated fat	35 g 3 g 0 mg 1 mg	Carbohydrate Fiber Cholesterol Sodium	2¹/₂ ¹/₂	Fruits & Vegetables Sugars	2	Fruit
p. 87 Grilled Fruit Kabobs ¹/₄ of recipe	126 Calories 1 g Protein 1 g Fat 0 g Saturated fat	32 g 4 g 0 mg 4 mg	Carbohydrate Fiber Cholesterol Sodium	2¹/₂ ¹/₂	Fruits & Vegetables Sugars	2	Fruit
p. 88 Amaretto & Almond-stuffed Peaches ¹/₄ of recipe	181 Calories 3 g Protein 8 g Fat 2 g Saturated fat	23 g 2 g 8 mg 30 mg	Carbohydrate Fiber Cholesterol Sodium	1 1 1¹/₂	Fruits & Vegetables Sugars Fats & Oils	1 ¹/₃ 1¹/₂	Fruit Other Carbohydrate Fat
p. 88 Poached Pears with Fruit Coulis ¹/₄ of recipe	134 Calories 1 g Protein 1 g Fat 0 g Saturated fat	34 g 8 g 0 mg 0 mg	Carbohydrate Fiber Cholesterol Sodium	2¹/₂	Fruits & Vegetables	1¹/₂	Fruit
p. 90 Old-fashioned Bread & Butter Pudding ¹/₄ of recipe	262 Calories 11 g Protein 9 g Fat 4 g Saturated fat	36 g 3 g 174 mg 275 mg	Carbohydrate Fiber Cholesterol Sodium	1 1 1 ¹/₂ ¹/₂ 1¹/₂	Starch Fruits & Vegetables Skim Milk Sugars Protein Fats & Oils	1 1 ¹/₂ ¹/₂ 1¹/₂	Starch Fruit Milk Skim Lean Meat Fat
p. 90 Apple & Plum Crumble ¹/₄ of recipe	326 Calories 8 g Protein 6 g Fat 1 g Saturated fat	66 g 10 g 0 mg 65 mg	Carbohydrate Fiber Cholesterol Sodium	2 1¹/₂ 1¹/₂ 1	Starch Fruits & Vegetables Sugars Fats & Oils	2 1 1 1	Starch Fruit Other Carbohydrate Fat

Recipe Name	Nutrient Information				Canadian Diabetes Association Food Choice Value		American Diabetes Association Exchanges	
p. 91 Black Forest Crepes $^1/_4$ of recipe (2 crepes)	256 9 g 9 g 4 g	Calories Protein Fat Saturated fat	35 g 1 g 66 mg 177 mg	Carbohydrate Fiber Cholesterol Sodium	$1^1/_2$ $^1/_2$ $^1/_2$ $^1/_2$ $1^1/_2$	Starch Fruits & Vegetables Sugars Protein Fats & Oils	$1^1/_2$ $^1/_3$ $^1/_3$ $^1/_2$ $1^1/_2$	Starch Fruit Other Carbohydrate Medium Fat Meat Fat
p. 92 Apricot & Apple Tarte Tatin $^1/_6$ of recipe	272 4 g 6 g 1 g	Calories Protein Fat Saturated fat	56 g 5 g 0 mg 169 mg	Carbohydrate Fiber Cholesterol Sodium	1 2 $1^1/_2$ 1	Starch Fruits & Vegetables Sugars Fats & Oils	1 $1^1/_2$ 1 1	Starch Fruit Other Carbohydrate Fat
p. 93 Chilled Lemon & Lime Mousse $^1/_4$ of recipe	366 6 g 23 g 14 g	Calories Protein Fat Saturated fat	34 g 0 g 79 mg 407 mg	Carbohydrate Fiber Cholesterol Sodium	$3^1/_2$ 1 4	Sugars Protein Fats & Oils	$2^1/_3$ 1 3	Other Carbohydrate High Fat Meat Fat
p. 95 Chocolate & Almond Custard Tart $^1/_8$ of recipe	212 6 g 10 g 3 g	Calories Protein Fat Saturated fat	27 g 1 g 54 mg 200 mg	Carbohydrate Fiber Cholesterol Sodium	1 1 $^1/_2$ $1^1/_2$	Starch Sugars Protein Fats & Oils	1 $^2/_3$ 2	Starch Other Carbohydrate Fat
p. 96 Lemon & Raisin Cheesecake with Cherries $^1/_8$ of recipe	249 10 g 8 g 3 g	Calories Protein Fat Saturated fat	35 g 1 g 13 mg 253 mg	Carbohydrate Fiber Cholesterol Sodium	1 $^1/_2$ $^1/_2$ 1 1 1	Starch Fruits & Vegetables 1% Milk Sugars Protein Fats & Oils	$1^1/_2$ $^1/_2$ $^1/_2$ $^1/_2$ $1^1/_2$	Starch Fruit Other Carbohydrate Very Lean Meat Fat
p. 96 Petits Coeurs à la Crème $^1/_4$ of recipe	155 8 g 6 g 3 g	Calories Protein Fat Saturated fat	19 g 1 g 21 mg 92 mg	Carbohydrate Fiber Cholesterol Sodium	1 1 $^1/_2$ $^1/_2$	2% Milk Sugars Protein Fats & Oils	$^1/_2$ $^2/_3$ $^1/_2$ $^1/_2$	Low Fat Milk Other Carbohydrate Protein Fat
p. 99 Raspberry & Blueberry Shortbread Stacks $^1/_4$ of recipe	412 5 g 21 g 12 g	Calories Protein Fat Saturated fat	53 g 3 g 53 mg 190 mg	Carbohydrate Fiber Cholesterol Sodium	2 1 1 4	Starch Fruits & Vegetables Sugars Fats & Oils	2 $^1/_3$ 1 4	Starch Fruit Other Carbohydrate Fat
p. 100 Raspberry & Ginger Sundaes $^1/_4$ of recipe	379 5 g 15 g 2 g	Calories Protein Fat Saturated fat	58 g 5 g 0 mg 468 mg	Carbohydrate Fiber Cholesterol Sodium	2 $2^1/_2$ 1 1 3	Starch Fruits & Vegetables 2% Milk Sugars Fats & Oils	2 $^1/_2$ $^1/_2$ $^1/_2$ $2^1/_2$	Starch Fruit Low Fat Milk Other Carbohydrate Fat

Recipe Name	Nutrient Information				Canadian Diabetes Association Food Choice Value		American Diabetes Association Exchanges	
p. 100 Exotic Fruit Salad with Cardamom $^1/_6$ of recipe	191 2 g 1 g 0 g	Calories Protein Fat Saturated fat	49 g 5 g 0 mg 5 mg	Carbohydrate Fiber Cholesterol Sodium	$3^1/_2$ 1	Fruits & Vegetables Sugars	2 1	Fruit Other Carbohydrate
p. 102 Banana Ice Cream with Chocolate & Hazelnut Topping $^1/_4$ of recipe	403 11 g 20 g 7 g	Calories Protein Fat Saturated fat	53 g 3 g 8 mg 151 mg	Carbohydrate Fiber Cholesterol Sodium	2 2 2 3	Fruits & Vegetables 2% Milk Sugars Fats & Oils	$1^1/_2$ 1 1 3	Fruit Low Fat Milk Other Carbohydrate Fat
p. 103 Summer Berry Frozen Dessert $^1/_4$ of recipe	161 5 g 2 g 1 g	Calories Protein Fat Saturated fat	33 g 5 g 5 mg 57 mg	Carbohydrate Fiber Cholesterol Sodium	1 1 $1^1/_2$	Fruits & Vegetables 1% Milk Sugars	$^1/_2$ $^1/_2$ 1	Fruit Very Low Fat Milk Other Carbohydrate
p. 103 Strawberry & Mascarpone Sorbet $^1/_4$ of recipe	341 7 g 23 g 20 g	Calories Protein Fat Saturated fat	30 g 2 g 5 mg 17 mg	Carbohydrate Fiber Cholesterol Sodium	$^1/_2$ 1 $1^1/_2$ 4	Fruits & Vegetables Whole Milk Sugars Fats & Oils	$^1/_3$ $^1/_2$ 1 4	Fruit Milk Whole Other Carbohydrate Fat
p. 106 Fruit Scones $^1/_{12}$ of recipe	78 2 g 2 g 0 g	Calories Protein Fat Saturated fat	14 g 1 g 0 mg 157 mg	Carbohydrate Fiber Cholesterol Sodium	1 $^1/_2$	Starch Fats & Oils	1 $^1/_2$	Starch Fat
p. 107 Grandma's Homemade Gingerbread $^1/_{16}$ of recipe	158 3 g 3 g 1 g	Calories Protein Fat Saturated fat	30 g 1 g 14 mg 182 mg	Carbohydrate Fiber Cholesterol Sodium	1 1 $^1/_2$ $^1/_2$	Starch Fruits & Vegetables Sugars Fats & Oils	1 $^1/_2$ $^1/_2$ $^1/_2$	Starch Fruit Other Carbohydrate Fat
p. 109 Date & Banana Loaf $^1/_{15}$ of recipe	126 3 g 1 g 0 g	Calories Protein Fat Saturated fat	29 g 2 g 15 mg 220 mg	Carbohydrate Fiber Cholesterol Sodium	1 1	Starch Fruits & Vegetables	1 $^2/_3$	Starch Fruit
p. 109 Fruit & Walnut Loaf $^1/_{18}$ of recipe	190 4 g 8 g 3 g	Calories Protein Fat Saturated fat	28 g 2 g 23 mg 131 mg	Carbohydrate Fiber Cholesterol Sodium	1 1 $1^1/_2$	Starch Fruits & Vegetables Fats & Oils	1 $^2/_3$ $1^1/_2$	Starch Fruit Fat
p. 110 Quick & Easy Swiss Roll $^1/_8$ of recipe	128 4 g 2 g 1 g	Calories Protein Fat Saturated fat	22 g 0 g 81 mg 110 mg	Carbohydrate Fiber Cholesterol Sodium	1 $^1/_2$ $^1/_2$	Starch Sugars Fats & Oils	1 $^1/_3$ $^1/_2$	Starch Other Carbohydrate Fat

Recipe Name	Nutrient Information				Canadian Diabetes Association Food Choice Value		American Diabetes Association Exchanges	
p. 111 Walnut Layer Cake 1/12 of recipe	257 6 g 12 g 3 g	Calories Protein Fat Saturated fat	32 g 1 g 43 mg 485 mg	Carbohydrate Fiber Cholesterol Sodium	1 1½ ½ 2	Starch Sugars Protein Fats & Oils	1 1 2½	Starch Other Carbohydrate Fat
p. 112 Carrot Cake 1/12 of recipe	137 4 g 3 g 1 g	Calories Protein Fat Saturated fat	26 g 3 g 5 mg 154 mg	Carbohydrate Fiber Cholesterol Sodium	1 1 ½	Starch Fruits & Vegetables Fats & Oils	1 2/3 ½	Starch Fruit Fat
p. 113 Orange & Almond Cake 1/10 of recipe	122 2 g 6 g 1 g	Calories Protein Fat Saturated fat	16 g 0 g 43 mg 173 mg	Carbohydrate Fiber Cholesterol Sodium	½ 1 1	Starch Sugars Fats & Oils	½ 2/3 1	Starch Other Carbohydrate Fat
p. 114 Rich Fruit Cake 1/20 of recipe	227 3 g 8 g 1 g	Calories Protein Fat Saturated fat	38 g 1 g 32 mg 99 mg	Carbohydrate Fiber Cholesterol Sodium	1 2 1½ 1	Starch Sugars Fats & Oils Extras	1 1⅓ 1½	Starch Other Carbohydrate Fat
p. 115 Mincemeat Tarts 1/12 of recipe	156 2 g 7 g 1 g	Calories Protein Fat Saturated fat	23 g 1 g 0 mg 143 mg	Carbohydrate Fiber Cholesterol Sodium	½ 1	Starch Fruits & Vegetables	½ 2/3 1	Starch Fruit Fat
p. 116 Peanut Butter & White Chocolate Cookies 1/25 of recipe	95 2 g 5 g 1 g	Calories Protein Fat Saturated fat	11 g 1 g 9 mg 45 mg	Carbohydrate Fiber Cholesterol Sodium	½ ½ 1	Starch Sugars Fats & Oils	½ 1/3 1	Starch Other Carbohydrate Fat
p. 117 Low-sugar Shortbread 1/8 of recipe	170 2 g 8 g 5 g	Calories Protein Fat Saturated fat	23 g 1 g 20 mg 74 mg	Carbohydrate Fiber Cholesterol Sodium	1 1 1½	Starch Sugars Fats & Oils	1 ½ 1½	Starch Other Carbohydrate Fat
p. 119 Cherry Almond Bars 1/16 of recipe	130 3 g 5 g 1 g	Calories Protein Fat Saturated fat	18 g 1 g 14 mg 106 mg	Carbohydrate Fiber Cholesterol Sodium	1 1 1	Starch Fats & Oils Extras	1 1	Starch Fat
p. 119 Fruity Flapjack Squares 1/25 of recipe	137 1 g 9 g 5 g	Calories Protein Fat Saturated fat	15 g 1 g 22 mg 81 mg	Carbohydrate Fiber Cholesterol Sodium	1 ½ 1½	Fruits & Vegetables Sugars Fats & Oils	2/3 1/3 1½	Fruit Other Carbohydrate Fat

Recipe Name	Nutrient Information				Canadian Diabetes Association Food Choice Value		American Diabetes Association Exchanges	
p. 120 Chocolate Brownies $^1/_{16}$ of recipe	121 3 g 5 g 1 g	Calories Protein Fat Saturated fat	17 g 2 g 27 mg 270 mg	Carbohydrate Fiber Cholesterol Sodium	1 1	Starch Fats & Oils	1 1	Starch Fat
p. 121 Easy Irish Soda Bread $^1/_{12}$ of recipe	153 6 g 2 g 0 g	Calories Protein Fat Saturated fat	30 g 4 g 1 mg 231 mg	Carbohydrate Fiber Cholesterol Sodium	$1^1/_2$ $^1/_2$ $^1/_2$	Starch Sugar Fats & Oils	$1^1/_2$ $^1/_2$	Starch Fat
p. 122 Farmhouse Whole-grain Bread $^1/_{15}$ of recipe	128 5 g 2 g 0 g	Calories Protein Fat Saturated fat	24 g 4 g 0 mg 35 mg	Carbohydrate Fiber Cholesterol Sodium	1 $^1/_2$ $^1/_2$	Starch Sugar Protein	$1^1/_3$	Starch

Index

Entries in italics denote variations on the main recipes

ACKNOWLEDGMENTS

Index and editorial assistance: Jessica Hughes
Nutritional analysis: Fiona Hunter
Production: Nigel Reed
North American Consultant:
Katherine E. Younker, MBA, RD, Certified Diabetes Educator